Obsessive-
Compulsive–
Related
Disorders

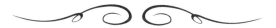

Obsessive-Compulsive-Related Disorders

Edited by
Eric Hollander, M.D.

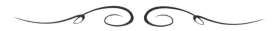

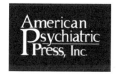

Washington, DC
London, England

Copyright © 1993 American Psychiatric Press, Inc.
ALL RIGHTS RESERVED
Manufactured in the United States of America on acid-free paper
First Edition

96 95 94 93 4 3 2 1

American Psychiatric Press, Inc.
1400 K Street, N.W., Washington, DC 20005

Library of Congress Cataloging-in-Publication Data
Obsessive-compulsive–related disorders / edited by Eric Hollander.
    p. cm.
    Includes bibliographical references and index.
    ISBN 0-88048-402-0
    1. Obsessive-compulsive disorder. I. Hollander, Eric, 1957– .
    [DNLM: 1. Obsessive-Compulsive Disorder. WM 176 01466]
RC533.029 1992
616.85′227—dc20
DNLM/DLC   92-10541
for Library of Congress   CIP

British Library Cataloguing in Publication Data
A CIP record is available from the British Library.

Contents

Contributors

Donna T. Anthony, M.D., Ph.D.
Instructor, Department of Psychiatry
College of Physicians and Surgeons
Columbia University
New York, New York

Elizabeth Brondolo, Ph.D.
Assistant Professor of Psychology
St. Johns University
Queens, New York

Emil F. Coccaro, M.D.
Associate Professor of Psychiatry
Medical College of Pennsylvania;
Director, Clinical Neuroscience Research Unit
Eastern Pennsylvania Psychiatric Institute
Philadelphia, Pennsylvania

Concetta M. DeCaria, M.S.
Coordinator, OCD Biological Studies Program
New York State Psychiatric Institute
New York, New York

Brian A. Fallon, M.D., M.P.H.
Instructor, Department of Psychiatry
College of Physicians and Surgeons
Columbia University
New York, New York

Eric Hollander, M.D.
Associate Professor of Clinical Psychiatry
College of Physicians and Surgeons
Columbia University;
Director, OCD Biological Studies Program
New York State Psychiatric Institute
New York, New York

L. K. George Hsu, M.D.
Associate Professor of Psychiatry
Western Psychiatric Institute and Clinic
University of Pittsburgh School of Medicine
Pittsburgh, Pennsylvania

Stephen C. Josephson, Ph.D.
Clinical Assistant Professor of Psychiatry (Psychology)
Cornell University College of Medicine
New York, New York

Zeev Kaplan, M.D.
Department of Psychiatry
Beer Sheva Mental Health Center
Beer Sheva, Israel

Richard J. Kavoussi, M.D.
Assistant Professor of Psychiatry
Medical College of Pennsylvania;
Clinical Neuroscience Research Unit
Eastern Pennsylvania Psychiatric Institute
Philadelphia, Pennsylvania

Walter H. Kaye, M.D.
Associate Professor of Psychiatry
University of Pittsburgh School of Medicine;
Director, Eating Disorder Module
Western Psychiatric Institute and Clinic
Pittsburgh, Pennsylvania

Seth Kindler, M.D.
Haim Sheba Medical Center
Division of Psychiatry
Tel Aviv University
Tel Aviv, Israel

Donald F. Klein, M.D.
Professor of Psychiatry
College of Physicians and Surgeons
Columbia University;
Director of Therapeutics and of Research Administration
New York State Psychiatric Institute
New York, New York

James F. Leckman, M.D.
Nelson Harris Professor of Child Psychiatry and Pediatrics
Child Study Center
Yale University School of Medicine
New Haven, Connecticut

Michael R. Liebowitz, M.D.
Professor of Clinical Psychiatry
College of Physicians and Surgeons
Columbia University;
Director of the Anxiety Clinic
New York State Psychiatric Institute
New York, New York

Katharine A. Phillips, M.D.
Instructor
Harvard Medical School;
Research Fellow, McLean Hospital
Boston, Massachusetts

Steven A. Rasmussen, M.D.
Associate Professor
Department of Psychiatry
Brown University Medical School;
Director, OCD Clinic
Butler Hospital
Providence, Rhode Island

Daniel J. Stein, M.B.
Instructor in Psychiatry
College of Physicians and Surgeons
Columbia University;
Research Fellow, OCD Biological Studies Program
New York State Psychiatric Institute
New York, New York

Susan E. Swedo, M.D.
Senior Research Staff
Child Psychiatry Branch
National Institute of Mental Health
Bethesda, Maryland

Theodore Weltzin, M.D.
Assistant Professor of Psychiatry
University of Pittsburgh School of Medicine;
Eating Disorder Module
Western Psychiatric Institute and Clinic
Pittsburgh, Pennsylvania

Joseph Zohar, M.D.
Professor of Psychiatry
Tel Aviv University;
Chairman, Division of Psychiatry
Haim Sheba Medical Center
Ramat Gan, Israel

Foreword

Given that in psychiatry we rarely know basic etiology, what do we mean when we say that disorders are related? The *categorical-vs.-dimensional* discussion, a common feature of nosological debate, should be understood as an ideological reflection of differences of opinion about the causal structure of psychiatric illness. The classic dimensional approach, as reflected in the use of the normal curve, is basically multicausal. In fact, one of the venerable derivations of the normal curve shows that it comes directly from the assumption that many simple causes are interacting in an additive way to produce an overall effect. In other words, the appearance of a dimensional relationship can actually be the manifestation of many discrete, additive causes.

Therefore, the distinction between the dimensional and the categorical approaches resolves into the distinction between multiple interacting causes and a single, often necessary, cause. The history of medicine has advanced through discoveries of disease entities that have corresponding typological regularities associated with them. Therefore, it is not surprising that such a traditional diagnostic approach should be part of medical psychiatric ideology. On the other hand, the history of applied psychology has consisted of the determination of certain quantitative measures, such as IQ, that have then been related in a linear fashion to validity criteria, such as school achievement. This position has resulted in the general attitude of psychologists that categories and diagnostic types are simply crude approximations of the underlying reality, useful only as terminological conveniences. That is, one may speak of tall people, average-sized people, and short people and get away with it for most purposes. However, if one is trying to develop comfortable chairs, one needs a refined measure, such as the inches scale, rather than coarse categories.

Such an approach, although entirely understandable, tends to prevent the detection of qualitative discontinuities. The fact that one may measure the size of all people with a foot rule does not imply that qualitative distinctions in height in such conditions as pituitary gigantism or cretinism do not exist.

This ideological controversy is derived from a basic biophobic-psychophobic antagonism. The "biophobes" refuse to admit the usefulness of categorizations that imply discrete etiologies as anything more than a crude approximation of the multifactorial interplay of variables that may be social, psychological, organic, etc. The "psychophobes" rely on discrete diagnostic categories in the hope that etiologic discovery will reveal the psychological and social factors to be ancillary epiphenomena. Even if one accepts a basically categorical approach, certain dimensions of variation, such as psychomotor activation or intelligence, cut across psychiatric subcategories. Therefore, even within subcategories, there may be variations that are relevant to both treatment and prognosis.[1]

Hollander (see Chapter 1) has drawn our attention to an apparently bipolar dimension that can descriptively rank various conditions. For instance, he posits a dimension of risk aversiveness as opposed to risk seeking, thus opposing OCD to borderline personality disorder. Is such a dimension, which closely resembles the harm-avoidance dimension of Cloninger, simply a useful, descriptive device, or is it indicative of some underlying relationship? Cloninger has hypothesized that this dimension reflects serotonergic activity.[2] For Cloninger, this ordered array of categories truly is the manifestation of an underlying rheostat-like contingency.

One of the nice things about dimensional thinking is that it lends itself to unifying hypotheses that cross categorical boundaries. As long as one thinks about a group of discrete categories, the relationships among these categories are purely nominal. Once one thinks in terms of ordering along a scale, new generalizations become possible and testable.

---

[1]Klein DF, Gittelman R, Quitkin F, et al: *Diagnosis and Drug Treatment of Psychiatric Disorders: Adults & Children,* 2nd Edition. Baltimore, MD, Williams & Wilkins, 1980.

[2]Cloninger CR: "A Systematic Method for Clinical Description and Classification of Personality Variants: A Proposal." *Archives of General Psychiatry* 44:573–588, 1987

Other descriptive dimensions seem more refractory to hypotheses. For instance, the cognitive-motoric dimension in which categories are ordered from purely obsessional to Tourette's syndrome may not indicate an underlying continuum but rather speak for quite different levels of pathophysiology. The dopamine-blocking drugs seem of value for treating Tourette's syndrome but are of no particular benefit for purely obsessional states. Rather than a dimension, this may represent a contrast of discrete mechanisms that may, to some degree, overlap.

There are ambiguities related to the uncertainty-certainty dimension. Delusional patients are certain when they should be uncertain, whereas patients with OCD are uncertain when they should be certain. We have hypothesized that this particular dimension might derive from malfunctioning of a neurophysiological, match-mismatch comparator that critically compares the high-level propositions we make about our life situation with incoming data. When the propositions and data are in harmony, we feel secure. When the data do not meet our propositions, we become uneasy. When there is a massive divergence, we may be driven to forming new propositions that subsume the divergent data. This propositional novelty is often accompanied by a sense of relief and an "Aha!" experience.

One can think of two ways the comparator might go wrong in measuring the gap between data and propositions. It might respond to a big gap as if there were no gap at all (e.g., a psychotic illumination), or it might misevaluate a small gap as if it were a big gap. This would result in maintained doubt about circumstances that the person understands should not engender doubt (e.g., Are my hands really clean?). In this case, the poles are opposing pathological ways of dealing with the gap between data and propositions. Because this complex match-mismatch device may have stabilizing negative feedback loops, one can easily posit a cybernetic pathology that would result in rapid oscillations in gap detection. This might be manifested in clinical fluctuations between obsessions and delusional convictions.

Are there dimensions that do not simply reflect the additive effect of many small causes but rather a smooth continuous increment of some underlying variable?

Outside of simple physical systems, in which variables such as temperature or voltage have a clear meaning, it is hard to find good examples of simple dimensionality. Much current pathophysiological speculation has centered about neurotransmitters. The reason is plain. Many of our cardinal drugs have very marked effects upon neurotransmitters. Therefore, it is easy to develop a variety of dimensional rheostat theories. The notion that depression came from too little norepinephrine and mania from too much sets the model for this field. It lends some inferential basis for a dimensional approach. Rather than coarse categories such as melancholia, dysthymia, normality, hypomania, and mania being erected, perhaps these categories reflect an underlying continuum of the amount of synaptic norepinephrine available. Serotonin has now replaced norepinephrine in the forefront of speculation.

The problem with such theories is that the same medications that have such powerful effects on patients with illnesses do remarkably little to "normal" persons. Although they experience the same norepinephrine reuptake blocking effects, normal subjects are not made manic by imipramine. I have suggested that our important psychotropic drugs work by the normalization of a deranged regulatory system, perhaps by repair of some cybernetic pathology such as the replacement of normal stabilizing negative feedback loops by positive feedback loops.[3] Such a cybernetic mishap can derive from either single major mishaps, which could nonetheless be manifested in an entire spectrum of psychopathology, or multiple incapacitations. One interesting model is provided by the recent work on cancer, which seems to indicate that the final formation of a malignancy depends upon multiple genetic inactivations. Crossing the malignancy threshold is due to a multicausal interaction that is patterned rather than additive.

It seems likely that the more stereotyped and homogeneous a disorder is, the better the chance of finding a convergence at one site in the pathophysiological chain. I have recently speculated that the

---

[3]Klein DF: "Cybernetics, Activation, and Drug Effects." *Acta Psychiatrica Scandinavica* 77:126–137, 1988.

spontaneous panic attack may often reflect a misfiring suffocation alarm.[4] Even if true, one could not assume that this misfiring was always due to the same causal network. Therefore, one possibility is to attempt to conceptualize psychopathological syndromes in terms of an intermediate level of structural pathology such as a displaced threshold or feedback loop. The resemblances between syndromes may not so much reflect common underlying etiology as much as similar derangements of adaptive mechanisms.

This may seem terminally vague. However, it does relate directly to the question of treatment because it is likely that our treatments are not hitting anywhere near the ultimate etiologies of our psychiatric illnesses, but rather are normalizing or compensating for adaptive derangements.

Let us put that aside for the moment. What are the types of evidence used to argue for relatedness? These types include

◆ Similarity of symptomatology
◆ Course
◆ Epidemiologic risk factors
◆ Frequent comorbidity
◆ Regular temporal transition from one syndrome to another
◆ Joint familial loading
◆ Specific responses to treatment
◆ Premorbid personality characteristics
◆ Sex ratio
◆ Age of onset
◆ Neurological deficits
◆ Psychological test performances
◆ Response to challenges
◆ Biochemical indices
◆ Neurological deficits
◆ Brain imaging patterns (both functional and anatomical)

---

[4]Klein DF: "False Suffocation Alarms, Spontaneous Panics, and Related Conditions: An Integrative Hypothesis." *Archives of General Psychiatry* (in press).

This partial, heterogeneous list indicates that we are looking at the distal manifestations of whatever has gone wrong in the hope that similarities will reveal process, and even causal, similarity.

Erecting categorical distinctions on the basis of differences in pharmacological reactivity is particularly persuasive when it is the more severe illness that responds best to a particular agent, as is the case in dissection of panic disorder from the general class of anxiety neurosis or of unipolar major depression and bipolar disorder from the general class of mood disorders.[5]

Pharmacological amalgamation is obviously a trickier affair because many active drugs have multiple effects. One would not want to assert that enuresis is a depressive equivalent because of its positive response to imipramine, although it would be worth investigating. In other words, pharmacological treatment resemblances, like all the other resemblances discussed, cannot definitively amalgamate. Clearly no indicator is definitive, but if several of these argued in unison, one's suspicions would have to be raised that some sort of relatedness is called for.

Grunbaum has emphasized the scientific utility of the notion of "consilience," in which a number of different aspects of a situation jump together to form a discernable pattern.[6] This is hypothesis formation rather than hypothesis testing, but one has to form them before one can test them.

However, even using a simple polygenic model, allowing for environmental interactions and phenocopies, the potential number of models that will fit any given factual situation proliferate to a daunting degree.

The attempt to determine whether other disorders are related to obsessive-compulsive disorder (OCD) is basically practical at this stage of our scientific development. OCD has been a notoriously

---

[5]Klein DF: "The Pharmacological Validation of Psychiatric Diagnosis," in *Validity of Psychiatric Diagnosis*. Edited by Robbins LN, Barrett N. New York, Raven, 1989, pp. 203–216.

[6]Grunbaum A: *The Foundations of Psychoanalysis: A Philosophical Critique*. Berkeley, CA, University of California Press, 1984

hard-to-treat syndrome. Recent studies of the pharmacotherapy and psychotherapy of OCD have provided reason for increasing optimism, although it is clear that we have not come as far in therapeutic efficacy as we have with panic disorder or major depression. It is not surprising that many would like to extend these therapeutic advances to the care of other difficult conditions. If the case can be made that these conditions are related to OCD, this heartens us to proceed with the difficult task of therapeutic trial and controlled evaluation, as well as gives us some direction concerning the sort of treatment likely to work. This book is a large step in that direction.

Donald F. Klein, M.D.

Acknowledgments

The editor acknowledges the guidance of Donald F. Klein, M.D., and Michael R. Liebowitz, M.D.

The editor also acknowledges scientific inspiration for the study of obsessive-compulsive–related disorders from Judith L. Rapoport, M.D., and Michael Jenike, M.D.

This work was funded in part by Research Scientist Development Award MH-00750 on the Psychobiology of Obsessive-Compulsive Related Disorders from the National Institute of Mental Health, Bethesda, M.D., to Dr. Hollander.

Chapter 1

Introduction

Eric Hollander, M.D.

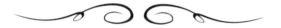

Obsessive-compulsive disorder (OCD) is a well-characterized syndrome classified in DSM-III-R (American Psychiatric Association 1987) as an anxiety disorder because obsessions are anxiety provoking and compulsions are anxiety reducing. Once considered a rare disorder, OCD is now known to be among the most common of psychiatric disorders. A number of trade books have recently brought this previously obscure disorder into the limelight and into the consciousness of the general population.[1]

While obsessions and compulsions are the sine qua non of OCD, obsessive thinking and compulsive rituals may also be found in other disorders. Because some of these disorders share certain common features, the notion of *obsessive-compulsive–related,* or spectrum, disorders has emerged.

These disorders are characterized by obsessive thoughts or pre-occupations with body appearance (body dysmorphic disorder), bodily sensations (depersonalization), body weight (anorexia ner-

---

[1] See, for example, Rapoport J: *The Boy Who Couldn't Stop Washing.* New York, Dutton, 1989.

vosa), or body illness (hypochondriasis); or by stereotyped, ritualistic, or driven behaviors such as tics (Tourette's syndrome), hair pulling (trichotillomania), sexual compulsions, pathological gambling, or other impulsive style disorders (see Figure 1–1). These common features suggest an overlap between OCD and somatoform (body dysmorphic disorder, hypochondriasis), dissociative (depersonalization), eating (anorexia nervosa), impulse dyscontrol (trichotillomania, pathological gambling, sexual compulsions), tic (Tourette's syndrome), impulsive personality (borderline), delusional (delusional

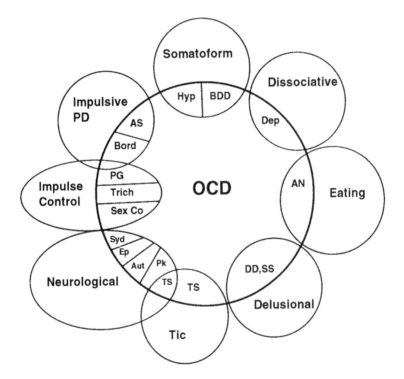

Figure 1–1. The spectrum of obsessive-compulsive–related disorders. Overlap between OCD and somatoform, dissociative, eating, delusional, tic, neurological, impulse control, and impulsive personality disorders. Abbreviations (clockwise from top): Hypochondriasis (Hyp); body dysmorphic disorder (BDD); depersonalization (Dep); anorexia nervosa (AN); delusional disorder, somatic subtype (DD,SS); Tourette's syndrome (TS); Parkinson's disease (Pk); autism (Aut); epilepsy (Ep); Sydenham's chorea (Syd); sexual compulsions (Sex Co); trichotillomania (Trich); pathological gambling (PG); borderline personality disorder (Bord); antisocial personality disorder (AS).

Table 1–1. Obsessive-compulsive–related disorders

Body dysmorphic disorder	Tourette's syndrome
Depersonalization disorder	Sexual compulsions
Anorexia nervosa	Pathological (compulsive) gambling
Hypochondriasis	Impulsive personality disorders
Trichotillomania	Delusional disorders

disorder, somatic subtype; schizophrenia), and neurological (Sydenham's chorea, parkinsonism, epilepsy, autism, pervasive developmental) disorders.

The disorders that will be examined for both similarities and differences with OCD are listed in Table 1–1.

While psychiatry primarily attempts to classify these disorders into categories, dimensional aspects of various spectrums may also be identified. One dimension may be conceptually defined by estimation of risk. This may include a *risk-aversive* (i.e., compulsive) end point with overestimation of the probability of future harm, and a *risk-seeking* (i.e., impulsive) end point involving action without full consideration of the negative consequences of behavior (Figure 1–2). Although many OCD patients are conceptualized as being near the compulsive, risk-aversive end of the spectrum, some OCD patients have considerably strong aggressive or sexual impulses, although

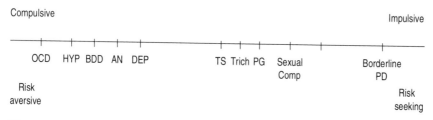

Figure 1–2. Dimensional aspects of the obsessive-compulsive–related disorder spectrum: risk-aversive/risk-seeking dimension. This dimension, from left to right, goes from "compulsive (risk aversive) disorders" to "mixed compulsive-impulsive disorders" to "impulsive (risk-seeking) disorders" as follows: obsessive-compulsive disorder (OCD), hypochondriasis (HYP), body dysmorphic disorder (BDD), anorexia nervosa (AN), depersonalization disorder (DEP), Tourette's syndrome (TS), trichotillomania (Trich), pathological gambling (PG), sexual compulsions (Sexual Comp), and borderline and antisocial personality disorders (Borderline PD).

often held in check. Disorders of impulse control, such as trichotillo-mania, pathological gambling, kleptomania, sexual "compulsions," and impulsive personality disorders (i.e., borderline personality disorder), may lie at the opposite extreme of this spectrum and involve underestimation of the negative consequences of impulsivity.

An alternative dimension ranges from cognitive (i.e., obsessional) features at one end point to motoric (i.e., ritualistic) behaviors at the other (Figure 1–3). Pure obsessions, hypochondriasis, depersonalization, and body dysmorphic disorder are primarily characterized by obsessive preoccupations. Childhood OCD, Tourette's syndrome, and trichotillomania are primarily characterized by motoric behavior.

Finally, a dimension ranging from obsessive uncertainty through overvalued ideas to delusional certainty may also exist (Figure 1–4). For example, OCD and body dysmorphic disorder include a well-defined subgroup of patients with transient delusional symptoms and considerable overvalued ideas. Schizophrenia and delusional disorder, somatic subtype may also include patients with prominent obsessive preoccupations. On the other hand, many OCD patients clearly articulate that their obsessions are not realistic and seem silly.

These *obsessive-compulsive–related disorders* (OCRDs) may share various characteristics, including

◆ Clinical symptoms
◆ Associated features such as age at onset, clinical course, family history, and comorbidity
◆ Presumed etiology (biology and neurology)

Figure 1–3. The cognitive-motoric dimension. This dimension, from left to right, goes from "disorders with primarily cognitive features" to "disorders with primarily motor features" as follows: purely obsessional, hypochondriasis (HYP), depersonalization disorder (DEP), body dysmorphic disorder (BDD), trichotillomania (Trich), childhood obsessive-compulsive disorder (OCD), and Tourette's syndrome (TS).

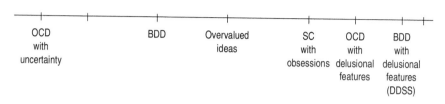

Figure 1–4. The uncertainty-certainty (delusional) dimension. This dimension, from left to right, goes from "disorders with prominent uncertainty (i.e., doubt)" to "disorders with premature certainty (i.e., delusions)" as follows: obsessive-compulsive disorder (OCD) with uncertainty, body dysmorphic disorder (BDD), overvalued ideas, schizophrenia (SC) with obsessions, OCD with delusional features, and body dysmorphic disorder with delusional features (delusional disorder, somatic subtype [DDSS]).

◆ Genetic/familial transmission
◆ Response to selective pharmacological or behavioral treatments

However, overlap between OCD and these various disorders on these features is not uniform. Although this overlap does not establish a definite relationship between disorders, it does provide confirmatory evidence to support a presumed relationship. Evidence for linkage of genetic/familial transmission may strongly suggest a relationship, as is found in Tourette's syndrome and OCD. This linkage, however, may explain only a small subgroup of the OCD population, because OCD is far more prevalent than is Tourette's syndrome.

Some of these disorders may share common biological and/or neurological markers, which may suggest a possible overlap in etiology. A careful history of prior infectious illness, head trauma, exposure to neurotoxins, hallucinogenic or psychotomimetic drugs, etc., may provide an important clue. New approaches such as the use of pharmacological challenges (i.e., *m*-chlorophenylpiperazine [m-CPP]) or imaging procedures (i.e., computed tomography, magnetic resonance imaging, positron-emission tomography) are of increasing importance in clarifying the relationship between different disorders.

Pharmacological dissection, as articulated by Donald F. Klein in the foreword to this book, may also support or discourage a relationship between diagnostic entities.

Obsessive-Compulsive Disorder

Before examining each of the related disorders, some critical discussion of the diagnostic, biological, and treatment (pharmacological and behavioral) issues of OCD itself is called for.

Once considered a rare disorder, OCD is now known to be among the most common of psychiatric disorders, with lifetime prevalence estimates of 2% to 3% of the population (Karno et al. 1988; Robins et al. 1984). However, these Epidemiologic Catchment Area estimates for community samples have been faulted by their inclusion of subjects with obsessive-compulsive symptoms of insufficient severity to meet DSM-III-R criteria for OCD. Thus, while 2% to 3% of the United States population have obsessive-compulsive symptoms, perhaps 1% to 2% would meet criteria for OCD. Patients with either obsessions or compulsions may meet criteria for OCD; however, over 90% of these subjects have both obsessions and compulsions (Rasmussen and Tsuang 1986). In the course of illness, perhaps 10% to 20% of OCD patients may manifest delusional conviction with regard to their obsessive-compulsive symptoms (Insel and Akiskal 1986). The prevalence of comorbid illnesses with OCD is very high. For example, approximately 80% of OCD patients may present with depressed mood, and 30% meet criteria for major affective disorder on admission (Rasmussen and Tsuang 1986).

Most biological models of OCD center around the role of serotonin (5-hydroxytryptamine [5-HT]) in the pathophysiology of the disorder. This model stems primarily from the finding that serotonin reuptake blockers such as clomipramine (DeVeaugh-Geiss et al. 1989), fluoxetine (Liebowitz et al. 1989; Pigott et al. 1990), and fluvoxamine (Goodman et al. 1989) are highly effective in the treatment of OCD, whereas other antidepressant medications such as desipramine (Zohar and Insel 1987) and clorgyline (Insel et al. 1983) are ineffective. These findings suggest that only a subset of antidepressant medications are effective in the treatment of OCD, and agents in this subgroup share serotonin reuptake blocking mechanisms. This model is supported by cerebrospinal fluid studies of the 5-HT metabolite 5-hydroxyindoleacetic acid (5-HIAA), the findings of which suggest elevated levels of 5-HIAA in OCD (Insel et al. 1985) or in a subgroup of OCD patients who are responsive to clomipramine (Thorén et al. 1980). Studies of peripheral 5-HT markers, such as 5-HT uptake and platelet imipramine binding, also document abnormalities, although findings between different groups have been somewhat mixed (Flament et al. 1987; Marazitti et al., in press; Weizman et al. 1986). Finally, pharmacological challenge studies with 5-HT agents such as m-CPP document behavioral hypersensitivity (Hollander et al. 1988; Zohar et al. 1987) and neuroendocrine blunting (Charney et al. 1988; Hollander et al. 1992; Zohar et al. 1987) in response to this partial 5-HT agonist. Successful treatment with serotonin reuptake blockers such as clomipramine (Zohar et al. 1988) and fluoxetine (Hollander et al. 1991a) can cause adaptive changes in both behavioral and neuroendocrine sensitivity, further suggesting a serotonergic role in both the disorder and the mechanism of treatment response.

However, clearly serotonin is not the only neurotransmitter that may play a role in this disorder. Noradrenergic mechanisms (suggested by clonidine challenge findings; see Hollander et al. 1988, 1991b) and dopaminergic mechanisms (suggested by symptom improvement in a subgroup of obsessive-compulsive patients with tics, schizotypal personality, and delusions following neuroleptic augmentation; see McDougle et al. 1990) may also play a role.

There is also evidence for neurological impairment underlying OCD in a subgroup of patients. Some patients manifest onset of illness following head trauma, encephalitis, or anoxia at birth, or in relationship to other neurological disorders such as Sydenham's chorea or Tourette's syndrome (Hollander et al. 1989a, 1991d). Others who remain refractory to pharmacological and behavioral treatment may obtain relief from current neurosurgical procedures and advances (Jenike et al. 1991a). Studies of neurological soft signs suggest subtle neurological dysfunction in a subgroup of OCD patients, consisting of fine-motor coordination, involuntary movement, and visuospatial deficits (Hollander et al. 1990b). These abnormalities may occur in the most severely obsessional patients and are often predictive of a poor outcome with serotonin reuptake blocker medications (Hollander et al. 1991c). Imaging studies have identified basal ganglia and orbital frontal cortical areas as regions of particular interest in the mediation of OCD symptoms as well as in the mediation of treatment response (Baxter et al. 1987; Swedo et al. 1989). Studies of biology and neurology in OCD reinforce the notion of heterogeneity with OCD and suggest that knowledge of an individual patient's biology may play a role in selecting the best available treatment (E. Hollander, C. M. DeCaria, J. B. Saoud, et al., unpublished manuscript, 1992).

It has now been established in a large series of double-blind, placebo-controlled trials that the potent and partially selective serotonin reuptake blocker clomipramine is effective in the treatment of OCD (DeVeaugh-Geiss et al. 1989). More selective serotonin reuptake blockers such as fluoxetine (Liebowitz et al. 1989; Pigott et al. 1990), fluvoxamine (Goodman et al. 1989), sertraline, and others also appear to be effective, although further large-scale double-blind, placebo-controlled studies are needed to document the efficacy of these treatments. Nevertheless, this class of medications appears to be effective in a substantial number of OCD patients: up to 60% of patients appear to be very much improved or much improved with chronic (8 to 12 weeks) therapeutic (high dose) treatment. However, up to 40% of patients remain refractory to this treatment approach. Even patients who are improved still suffer from obsessions and compulsions, although they may be considerably less disabled from the symptoms. Attempts at augmentation of antiobsessional treatments may result in additional improvements for some patients (Hollander et al. 1990a; Jenike et al. 1991b; Markovitz et al. 1990). In addition, we do not speak of a cure, but rather a partial remission of symptoms, which often recur upon discontinuation of treatment (Pato et al. 1988).

Likewise for behavioral therapies for OCD, a substantial number of patients may achieve considerable improvement with exposure and response-prevention techniques (Foa and Steketee 1989). However, most studies of behavior therapy do not include patients who are not capable or willing to expose themselves to situations that cause obsessional concern or to attempt to resist their compulsions. Thus, completers of the protocol are almost always by definition improved, and the large number of dropouts are often not included in the data analysis. In addition, depressed patients, those without clear-cut rituals, those with pure obsessions or slowness, and those with comorbid Axis II disorders such as schizotypal personality disorder often have a poor outcome with behavior therapy.

Treatment studies of the OCRDs are even less well characterized overall than those of OCD. For the most part, they consist of open clinical series, and large-scale placebo-controlled studies are lacking. However, by conceptualizing OCRDs as a group of related disorders, the hope is to generate the large-scale diagnostic, biological, and treatment studies needed to definitively characterize this spectrum of fascinating disorders. The clinical resemblance between these disorders is heartening and suggests the need to extend these pilot studies of antiobsessional treatments to other related disorders.

However, response to antiobsessional treatments is not sufficient to document a link between disorders. For example, response to serotonin reuptake blockers does not define the OCRDs, because disorders such as depression, panic disorder, and social phobia may respond to this treatment. Nonetheless, a preferential response to serotonin rather than norepinephrine reuptake blockers, coupled with symptomatic and biological overlap, may define the spectrum.

Pharmacological Dissection of Impulsivity and Compulsivity

As noted above, *impulsive*-style disorders may be phenomenologically distinguished from *compulsive*-style disorders. For individuals with impulsive-style disorders some pleasurable aspects are derived from the impulsive behavior, whereas for individuals with compulsive-style disorders the compulsive behavior is tension reducing but not pleasurable. At times, the distinction between tension-reducing behavior and pleasure-generating behavior is not clear-cut.

Pharmacological challenge studies also reinforce the distinction between impulsive and compulsive disorders. Our pilot challenge studies with the partial 5-HT agonist m-CPP (0.5 mg/kg po) suggest behavioral and neuroendocrine differences between impulsive and compulsive disorders. OCD, Tourette's syndrome, and eating disorder patients with prominent obsessional features experience exacerbation of obsessive symptoms in response to m-CPP. However, impulsive personality (i.e., borderline) patients not only fail to develop obsessive or dysphoric symptoms, but also experience a sense of "high" following m-CPP. In terms of neuroendocrine responsivity, OCD, Tourette's syndrome, and eating disorder patients show prolactin blunting in response to m-CPP challenge, whereas subjects with borderline personality disorder and normal subjects have a robust rise in prolactin in response to m-CPP.

Drug treatment studies also suggest pharmacological dissection between impulsivity and compulsivity. Compulsive-style disorders such as OCD, body dysmorphic disorder, hypochondriasis, depersonalization disorder, and anorexia nervosa respond preferentially to serotonin reuptake blocker medications. However, it remains to be seen whether impulsive-style disorders, such as pathological gambling, sexual compulsions, and paraphilias, and impulsive-style personality disorders have an equal responsivity to this treatment approach. For example, sexual obsessions, a typical subtype of OCD, are highly responsive to serotonin reuptake blocker treatment, whereas paraphilias and sexual impulsions appear less responsive to this treatment. Trichotillomania, which has both compulsive and impulsive qualities, may have an intermediate response, with good initial response but unclear long-term outcome to this treatment.

The Obsessive-Compulsive–Related Disorders

Hollander and Phillips, in Chapter 2, suggest that body image and experience disorders are not generally conceptualized as being related to OCD. However, these disorders involve obsessive preoccupation with the body and its relationship to the world, may have premorbid obsessional traits and similar associated features, and seem to have a preferential response to the serotonin reuptake blockers.

In Chapter 3, Kaye and colleagues have demonstrated that anorexia nervosa patients have multiple obsessive and compulsive symptoms of a severity equal to that seen in OCD patients. Evidence for similar serotonergic dysregulation in anorexia and OCD is suggested by increased cerebrospinal fluid 5-HIAA in both disorders. The behavioral hypersensitivity (Buttinger et al. 1990) and neuroendocrine blunting (Brewerton et al. 1989) in response to the partial 5-HT agonist m-CPP in eating disorder patients with obsessional features parallel similar findings in OCD (Hollander et al. 1992). Again, there appears to be a preferential response to the serotonin reuptake blockers.

Fallon and co-workers, in Chapter 4, describe a subtle distinction between OCD and hypochondriasis. Whereas many OCD patients are fearful of developing an illness, hypochondriacal patients are fearful that they are already ill. Nevertheless, there is considerable symptomatic overlap, and preliminary evidence suggests a preferential response to the serotonin reuptake blockers.

In Chapter 5, Swedo describes trichotillomania as a pathological grooming behavior. The motoric/compulsive nature of this disorder and its lack of cognitive/obsessional features are described. Relatively high rates of impulsive-style personality disorders are found within trichotillomanic patients. Perhaps this might contribute to the subtle distinctions found between the neurobiology of trichotillomania and OCD. Although serotonin reuptake blockers are effective in short-term trials, long-term outcome is not clear with these agents, and other agents such as lithium that are effective for impulsivity may also be efficacious. Perhaps future trials will address the impulsive and motoric features of trichotillomania.

The phenomenology, course, neurobiology, and treatment of Tourette's syndrome have been described by Leckman in Chapter 6. The genetic and familial link between OCD and Tourette's syndrome appears very convincing. Furthermore, considerable difficulty sometimes occurs in distinguishing between tics, compulsions, and impulsions, all of which may be characteristic of Tourette's syndrome. This difficulty suggests that considerable conceptual and methodological issues must be addressed in studies of the link between Tourette's syndrome and OCD (Hollander et al. 1989b). Although there is considerable overlap in neurological and neuropsychological markers between Tourette's syndrome and OCD, serotonergic tone may differ, which may reflect the compulsive nature of OCD and the impulsive nature of Tourette's syndrome (Hollander et al. 1989b).

Anthony and Hollander, in Chapter 7, describe sexual obsessions and compulsions. Sexual obsessions may represent a true subtype of OCD and appear to respond accordingly. Sexual compulsions involve a pleasurable element and may be more akin to impulsive and addictive disorders. Preliminary evidence suggests pharmacological dissection between the compulsive and impulsive sexual disorders.

In Chapter 8, DeCaria and Hollander describe the clinical features and course of illness of pathological (i.e., compulsive) gambling, a devastating illness with impulsive, compulsive, and addictive features. Further work is needed on the biological basis and treatment outcome of this relatively neglected illness that is characterized by both compulsive and impulsive features.

The spectrum of impulsive personality disorders and disorders of impulse control is discussed by Kavoussi and Coccaro in Chapter 9. Although there is evidence for marked differences in the biology of serotonergic function between the impulsive and compulsive disorders, serotonin reuptake blockers may be effective in the treatment of some patients on both ends of the spectrum. This puzzling finding reinforces the link between these disorders. It also suggests that serotonin reuptake blockers, rather than increasing or decreasing serotonergic tone, may work to stabilize this system.

In Chapter 10, Zohar and colleagues describe the overlap of delusional symptoms in OCD and obsessive symptoms in psychotic disorders. Rather than being limited by categorical diagnoses, the authors emphasize the need to diagnose and treat symptom clusters, an approach that may lead to several important developments.

Josephson and Brondolo, in Chapter 11, demonstrate that specific behavioral techniques that are effective in treating obsessions and compulsions in OCD may also have an important role in the treatment of many of the OCRDs. This finding also has important diagnostic implications with regard to the notion of the spectrum of OCRDs.

Finally, in Chapter 12, Stein and Hollander review the obsessive-compulsive–related spectrum of disorders along both categorical and dimensional models. This approach may have important implications for the way we conceptualize disorders and diagnose and treat patients who suffer from this often puzzling group of disorders of rapidly growing importance.

References

American Psychiatric Association: Diagnostic and Statistical Manual of Mental Disorders, 3rd Edition, Revised. Washington, DC, American Psychiatric Association, 1987

Baxter LR Jr, Phelps ME, Mazziotta JC, et al: Local cerebral glucose metabolic rates in obsessive-compulsive disorder: a comparison with rates in unipolar depression and in normal controls. Arch Gen Psychiatry 44:211–218, 1987

Brewerton T, Murphy D, Jimerson DC: A comparison of neuroendocrine responses to L-TRP and m-CPP in bulimics and controls. Biol Psychiatry 25 (no 7A, suppl):19A, 1989

Buttinger K, Hollander E, Walsh BT: m-CPP challenges in eating disorder patients. Paper presented at the 143rd annual meeting of the American Psychiatric Association, New York, NY, May 1990

Charney DS, Goodman WK, Price LH, et al: Serotonin function in obsessive-compulsive disorder: a comparison of the effects of tryptophan and m-chlorophenylpiperazine in patients and healthy subjects. Arch Gen Psychiatry 45:177–185, 1988

DeVeaugh-Geiss J, Landau P, Katz R: Treatment of obsessive compulsive disorder with clomipramine. Psychiatric Annals 19:97–101, 1989

Flament MF, Rapoport JL, Murphy DL, et al: Biochemical changes during clomipramine treatment of childhood obsessive-compulsive disorder. Arch Gen Psychiatry 44:219–225, 1987

Foa E, Steketee G: Obsessive-compulsive disorder, in Handbook of Phobia Therapy: Rapid Symptom Relief in Anxiety Disorders. Edited by Lindemann C. Northvale, NJ, Jason Aronson, 1989, pp 181–206

Goodman WK, Price LH, Rasmussen SA, et al: Efficacy of fluvoxamine in obsessive-compulsive disorder: a double-blind comparison with placebo. Arch Gen Psychiatry 46:36–44, 1989

Hollander E, Fay M, Cohen B, et al: Serotonergic and noradrenergic sensitivity in obsessive-compulsive disorder: behavioral findings. Am J Psychiatry 145:1015–1017, 1988

Hollander E, DeCaria C, Liebowitz MR: Biological aspects of obsessive compulsive disorder. Psychiatric Annals 19:80–87, 1989a

Hollander E, Liebowitz MR, DeCaria CM: Conceptual and methodological issues in studies of obsessive-compulsive disorder and Tourette's disorders. Psychiatr Dev 7:267–296, 1989b

Hollander E, DeCaria CM, Schneier FR, et al: Fenfluramine augmentation of serotonin reuptake blockade antiobsessional treatment. J Clin Psychiatry 51:119–123, 1990a

Hollander E, Schiffman E, Cohen B, et al: Signs of central nervous system dysfunction in obsessive-compulsive disorder. Arch Gen Psychiatry 47:27–32, 1990b

Hollander E, DeCaria C, Gully R, et al: Effects of chronic fluoxetine treatment on behavioral and neuroendocrine responses to meta-chloro-phenylpiperazine in obsessive-compulsive disorder. Psychiatry Res 36:1–17, 1991a

Hollander E, DeCaria C, Nitescu A, et al: Noradrenergic function in obsessive-compulsive disorder: behavioral and neuroendocrine responses to clonidine and comparison to healthy controls. Psychiatry Res 37:161–177, 1991b

Hollander E, DeCaria CM, Saoud JB, et al: Neurological soft signs in obsessive-compulsive disorder (letter in reply to Bihari et al). Arch Gen Psychiatry 48:278–279, 1991c

Hollander E, Liebowitz MR, Rosen WT: Neuropsychiatric and neuropsychological studies in obsessive-compulsive disorder, in Psychobiology of Obsessive-Compulsive Disorder. Edited by Zohar J, Insel TR, Rasmussen S. New York, Springer, 1991d, pp 126–145

Hollander E, DeCaria CM, Nitescu A, et al: Serotonergic function in obsessive-compulsive disorder: behavioral and neuroendocrine responses to oral m-chlorophenylpiperazine and fenfluramine in patients and healthy volunteers. Arch Gen Psychiatry 49:21–28, 1992

Insel TR, Akiskal HS: Obsessive-compulsive disorder with psychotic features: a phenomenologic analysis. Am J Psychiatry 143:1527–1533, 1986

Insel TR, Murphy DL, Cohen RM, et al: Obsessive-compulsive disorder: a double-blind trial of clomipramine and clorgyline. Arch Gen Psychiatry 40:605–612, 1983

Insel TR, Mueller EA, Alterman I, et al: Obsessive-compulsive disorder and serotonin: is there a connection? Biol Psychiatry 20:1174–1188, 1985

Jenike MA, Baer L, Ballantine HT, et al: Cingulotomy for refractory obsessive-compulsive disorder: a long-term follow-up of 33 patients. Arch Gen Psychiatry 48:548–555, 1991a

Jenike MA, Baer L, Buttolph L: Buspirone augmentation of fluoxetine in patients with obsessive compulsive disorder. J Clin Psychiatry 52:13–14, 1991b

Karno M, Golding JM, Sorenson SB, et al: The epidemiology of obsessive-compulsive disorder in five US communities. Arch Gen Psychiatry 45:1094–1099, 1988

Liebowitz MR, Hollander E, Schneier F, et al: Fluoxetine treatment of obsessive-compulsive disorder: an open clinical trial. J Clin Psychopharmacol 9:423–427, 1989

Marazitti D, Hollander E, Lensi P, et al: Peripheral markers of serotonin and dopamine function in obsessive-compulsive disorder. Psychiatry Res (in press)

Markovitz PJ, Stagno SJ, Calabrese JR: Buspirone augmentation of fluoxetine in obsessive-compulsive disorder. Am J Psychiatry 147:798–800, 1990

McDougle CJ, Goodman WK, Price LH, et al: Neuroleptic addition in fluvoxamine-refractory obsessive-compulsive disorder. Am J Psychiatry 147:652–654, 1990

Pato MT, Zohar-Kadouch R, Zohar J, et al: Return of symptoms after discontinuation of clomipramine in patients with obsessive-compulsive disorder. Am J Psychiatry 145:1521–1525, 1988

Pigott TA, Pato MT, Bernstein SE, et al: Controlled comparisons of clomipramine and fluoxetine in the treatment of obsessive-compulsive disorder: behavioral and biological results. Arch Gen Psychiatry 47:926–932, 1990

Rasmussen SA, Tsuang MT: Clinical characteristics and family history in DSM-III obsessive-compulsive disorder. Am J Psychiatry 143:317–322, 1986

Robins LN, Helzer JE, Weissman MM, et al: Lifetime prevalence of specific psychiatric disorders in three sites. Arch Gen Psychiatry 41:949–958, 1984

Swedo SE, Schapiro MB, Grady CL, et al: Cerebral glucose metabolism in childhood-onset obsessive-compulsive disorder. Arch Gen Psychiatry 46:518–523, 1989

Thorén P, Åsberg M, Bertilsson L, et al: Clomipramine treatment of obsessive-compulsive disorder, II: biochemical aspects. Arch Gen Psychiatry 37:1289–1294, 1980

Weizman A, Carmi M, Hermesh H, et al: High-affinity imipramine binding and serotonin uptake in platelets of eight adolescent and ten adult obsessive-compulsive patients. Am J Psychiatry 143:335–339, 1986

Zohar J, Insel TR: Obsessive-compulsive disorder: psychobiological approaches to diagnosis, treatment, and pathophysiology. Biol Psychiatry 22:667–687, 1987

Zohar J, Mueller EA, Insel TR, et al: Serotonergic responsivity in obsessive-compulsive disorder: comparison of patients and healthy controls. Arch Gen Psychiatry 44:946–951, 1987

Zohar J, Insel TR, Zohar-Kadouch RC, et al: Serotonergic responsivity in obsessive-compulsive disorder: effects of chronic clomipramine treatment. Arch Gen Psychiatry 45:167–172, 1988

Chapter 2

Body Image and Experience Disorders

Eric Hollander, M.D.
Katharine A. Phillips, M.D.

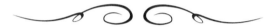

Persons' image or experience of their body may go awry in various ways. For example, they may become preoccupied with their appearance, or they may experience their body, or sensations from within their body, as altered in some way. These experiences form the core symptoms of *body dysmorphic disorder* (BDD) and *depersonalization disorder* (DEP). A hallmark and common organizing principle of both disorders is an obsessive preoccupation, either with imagined body defects or with perceived body sensory alterations, often coupled with compulsive checking behaviors. Thus, from a clinical standpoint, these disorders may be related to OCD and are here discussed together.

According to DSM-III-R (American Psychiatric Association 1987), BDD is classified as a somatoform disorder, DEP as a dissociative disorder, and obsessive-compulsive disorder (OCD) as an anxiety disorder. However, few systematic reports clearly support the existence of BDD or DEP as independent diagnostic entities. In this

Supported in part by Research Scientist Development Award MH-00750 (to Dr. Hollander) from the National Institute of Mental Health, Bethesda, Maryland.

chapter we will explore and contrast 1) symptomatic overlap, 2) associated features, 3) presumed etiology, and 4) treatment response of BDD, DEP and OCD.

Diagnostic Features

Body Dysmorphic Disorder

Body dysmorphic disorder is defined by DSM-III-R as a preoccupation with some imagined defect in appearance in a normal-appearing person (see Table 2–1). Common complaints involve facial flaws. If a slight physical anomaly is present, the person's concern is grossly excessive. The belief in the defect is not of delusional intensity, as in delusional disorder, somatic type (DDST), and it does not occur exclusively during the course of anorexia nervosa or transexualism (DSM-III-R). Other partially overlapping terms for BDD include *dysmorphophobia* and *monosymptomatic hypochondriasis.*

Case 1: Body Dysmorphic Disorder

A 25-year-old single white male initially became ill during high school, and this illness worsened upon his entering college. He was preoccupied with a perceived abnormality in the width of his nose. He frequently felt compelled to check his appearance in the mirror, and when this confirmed his perceived defect, he became very upset and anxious. He often tensed his face in an attempt to make his nose appear narrower. He became reluctant to socialize or attend classes because of his extreme self-consciousness about his nose. At times he could acknowledge that his mind was playing tricks on him, but at other times he was certain that the defect was real. Secondary to this obsessive fixation on his nose, the patient became increasingly anxious and depressed. He developed neurovegetative symptoms of major depression that failed to respond to insight-oriented psychotherapy or therapeutic trials of imipramine and, later, phenelzine. He was hospitalized and treated with ECT, with subsequent improvement in his depression but no resolution of his BDD. Subsequent therapeutic trials with tricyclics, monoamine oxidase (MAO) inhibi-

Table 2–1.	Comparison of DSM-III-R diagnostic criteria for body dysmorphic disorder; obsessive-compulsive disorder; delusional disorder, somatic type; and hypochondriasis

Body dysmorphic disorder (300.70)

A. Preoccupation with some imagined defect in appearance in a normal-appearing person. If a slight physical anomaly is present, person's concern is grossly excessive.

B. The belief in the defect is not of delusional intensity, as in delusional disorder, somatic type (i.e., the person can acknowledge the possibility that he or she may be exaggerating the extent of the defect or that there may be no defect at all).

C. Occurrence not exclusively during the course of anorexia nervosa or transsexualism.

Obsessive-compulsive disorder (300.30) (only criteria for obsessions listed)

A. Either obsessions or compulsions.

Obsessions: (1), (2), (3), and (4)

1. Recurrent and persistent ideas, thoughts, impulses, or images that are experienced, at least initially, as intrusive and senseless, e.g., a parent's having repeated impulses to kill a loved child, a religious person's having recurrent blasphemous thoughts.

2. The person attempts to ignore or suppress such thoughts or impulses or to neutralize them with some other thought or action.

3. The person recognizes that the obsessions are the product of his or her own mind, not imposed from without (as in thought insertion).

4. If another Axis I disorder is present, the content of the obsession is unrelated to it . . .

B. The obsessions [or compulsions] cause marked distress, are time-consuming (take more than an hour a day), or significantly interfere with the person's normal routine, occupational functioning, or usual social activities or relationships with others.

Delusional disorder, somatic type (297.10) (delusional disorder in which the predominant theme of the delusion(s) is that the person has some physical defect, disorder, or disease)

A. Nonbizarre delusion(s) (i.e., involving situations that occur in real life, such as being followed, poisoned, infected, loved at a distance, having a disease, being deceived by one's spouse or lover) of at least 1 month's duration.

B. Auditory or visual hallucinations, if present, are not prominent . . .

C. Apart from the delusion(s) or its ramifications, behavior is not obviously odd or bizarre.

D. If a major depressive or manic syndrome has been present during the delusional disturbance, the total duration of all episodes of the mood syndrome has been brief relative to the total duration of the delusional disturbance.

E. Has never met criterion A for schizophrenia, and it cannot be established that an organic factor initiated and maintained the disturbance.

Table 2–1.	Comparison of DSM-III-R diagnostic criteria for body dysmorphic disorder; obsessive-compulsive disorder; delusional disorder, somatic type; and hypochondriasis *(continued)*

Hypochondriasis (300.70)

A. Preoccupation with the fear of having, or the belief that one has, a serious disease, based on the person's interpretation of physical signs or sensations as evidence of physical illness.

B. Appropriate physical evaluation does not support the diagnosis of any physical disorder that can account for the physical signs or sensations or the person's unwarranted interpretation of them, **and** the symptoms in A are not just symptoms of panic attacks.

C. The fear of having, or the belief that one has, a disease persists despite medical reassurance.

D. Duration of the disturbance is at least 6 months.

E. The belief in A is not of delusional intensity, as in delusional disorder, somatic type (i.e., the person can acknowledge the possibility that his or her fear of having, or belief that he or she has, a serious disease is unfounded).

Source. Reprinted with permission from American Psychiatric Association *Diagnostic and Statistical Manual of Mental Disorders,* 3rd Edition, Revised. Washington, DC, American Psychiatric Association, 1987, pp. 202–203, 247, 256, 261. Copyright 1987, American Psychiatric Association.

tors, benzodiazepines, neuroleptics, and anticonvulsants were without effect on his BDD symptoms.

After discharge from the hospital, he saw a plastic surgeon, who performed a rhinoplasty. This caused considerable relief that lasted for 2 years. However, he then became focused on his left testicle. He experienced uncomfortable sensations in this region, and on examining himself in a mirror, his left testicle appeared to hang higher than his right testicle. He again saw a surgeon, who performed surgery on his left testicle to correct this perceived defect and to repair a hydrocele. This resulted in considerable relief for $1\frac{1}{2}$ years.

However, he once again became preoccupied with his appearance, this time with his buttocks. When wearing pants, he experienced chafing of his buttocks that resulted in severe discomfort. Because of the perceived defect in the shape of his buttocks and the resulting physical discomfort resulting from wearing pants, he refused to socialize. He was more comfortable wearing sweat pants, which did not have a seam down the middle, or shorts. He frequently checked himself in the mirror, and he became convinced that he saw fatty deposits in his buttocks. Again, he consulted a surgeon, who performed liposuction to remove the imagined fatty deposits. When told that he would have bruising and swelling for 6 months following the operation, he no longer was preoccupied with his buttocks, and successfully completed his undergraduate education. However, when the 6 months elapsed and the problem with his buttocks persisted, he once again relapsed.

Treatment consisted of a 12-week trial of clomipramine, 250 mg/day, which resulted in a moderate, but not complete, improvement in body dysmorphic symptoms and mood. Augmentation with buspirone, 50 mg/day, resulted in his being very much improved. This improvement has continued for 1 year of follow-up.

Depersonalization Disorder

The essential feature of DEP, according to DSM-III-R, is the occurrence of persistent or recurrent episodes of depersonalization sufficiently severe to cause marked distress. The symptom of depersonalization involves alteration in the perception or experience of the self in which the usual sense of one's own reality is temporarily lost or changed. This is manifested by a feeling of detachment from, or being an outside observer of, one's mental processes or body, or of feeling like an automaton or as if in a dream. Various types of sensory anesthesia and a sensation of not being in complete control of one's actions, including speech, are often present. All of these feelings are ego-dystonic, and the person maintains intact reality testing.

Case 2: Depersonalization Disorder

A 23-year-old professional became ill with the flu for 2 weeks. Following this illness, he became obsessed with the possibility that he had developed AIDS. This thought persisted for 2 months, and he became progressively more anxious and fearful of dying. He then had a sudden onset of visual changes and perceived the outside world to be altered, as if in a fog. Things seemed strangely two-dimensional. His thinking became slower, and he felt emotionally flat, unable to experience any emotions such as fear, anxiety, or happiness. He felt detached from his body; he had melting sensations in his body and twitching and heaviness in his head. He developed considerable difficulty with visuospatial tasks, such as drawing and reading maps, and he got lost in hallways. He did not meet the criteria for a major depressive disorder.

The patient's premorbid history revealed long-term perfectionistic and obsessional traits. He had previously felt his nose was misshapen and had disliked his physical appearance and hair. Six years earlier, he had had a similar transient episode of derealization following ingestion of hallucinogenic mushrooms. Five years previously, he had had an episode of major depression following a romantic rejection characterized by hopelessness and reversed vegetative features. Family history was significant for pathological gambling and affective disorder in first-degree relatives.

Therapeutic trials with lithium, tranylcypromine, lorazepam, and carbamazepine were without effect. The patient's symptoms persisted for 2 years, and he became unable to function in his job because he was constantly monitoring his altered perceptions. He consulted several medical specialists and had a number of diagnostic procedures. A magnetic resonance imaging (MRI) was normal, but a single-photon emission computed tomography (SPECT) scan suggested decreased metabolic activity in the left caudate and nonspecific heterogeneous activity bilaterally in the posterior frontal lobes. Neurometric brain mapping revealed diffuse increased alpha-activity, abnormal left anterior and posterior temporal lobe theta activity, and left temporal and frontal abnormalities on auditory and visual evoked potentials. Neurological soft-sign examination revealed no abnormal soft signs. Neuropsychological testing revealed average to above-average intelligence and slow and accurate performance on visuospatial tasks such as the Matching Familiar Figures test. [These findings are of interest and are reminiscent of findings in OCD such as frontal and caudate abnormalities on SPECT, excess alpha and theta activity on topographic electroencephalogram, and slow and accurate performance on visuospatial testing.]

The patient was treated with fluoxetine, 80 mg/day, which was subsequently augmented with buspirone, 60 mg/day. After 12 weeks he had substantial improvement in his visual abnormalities and detached feelings. He began to perceive the world in three dimensions and was able to experience emotions again. He began a fulfilling relationship with a woman and returned to work, on which he was now able to concentrate and focus.

Obsessive-Compulsive Disorder

Obsessive-compulsive disorder is defined in DSM-III-R as the presence of either obsessions or compulsions that cause marked distress, are time consuming, or significantly interfere with functioning. Obsessions are defined as persistent ideas, thoughts, impulses, or images that are experienced, at least initially, as intrusive or senseless. This definition could conceivably include patients with BDD or DEP.

Diagnostic Issues

Research on BDD and DEP is still in an early stage, with no existing large controlled studies of BDD or DEP, nor comparisons of these disorders with OCD. The bulk of the literature consists of anecdotal case reports and a few analogue studies in nonclinical populations.

Body Dysmorphic Disorder

Current diagnostic issues in BDD center around the following: 1) Is BDD a discrete syndrome, and does primary BDD differ from secondary BDD? and 2) What are the boundaries of BDD with "normal" concern with appearance?

The relationship between BDD and other disorders, notably DDST, and OCD will be discussed later in this chapter. Phillips and Hollander (in press) have recently reviewed these diagnostic controversies for BDD in the upcoming *DSM-IV Source Book*.

Is BDD a discrete syndrome?   Early reports suggested that BDD, or dysmorphophobia, was a distinct symptom cluster in some patients requesting cosmetic surgery (Andreasen and Bardach 1977; Thomas 1984). However, Munro and Stewart (1991) have pointed out that pathological conviction of body abnormalities may occur in several disorders, including OCD, personality disorders, somatoform disorders, schizophrenia, affective illness, and organic mental disorders. Thomas (1984) suggested that "dysmorphophobia" be applied only to patients without any of these other psychiatric illnesses and that the term "secondary, or symptomatic, dysmorphophobia" be used when another mental illness was present. However, others have suggested that the distinction between primary and secondary dysmorphophobia is arbitrary and that both conditions respond to similar treatments (Hollander et al. 1990a; Phillips et al., in press).

What are the boundaries of BDD with normal concern with appearance? Surveys of college student populations suggest that up to 70% are dissatisfied with some aspect of their bodies, 46% are preoccupied with this aspect of their appearance, 48% exaggerate their perceived body image, and 28% do all three (Fitts et al. 1989). These symptoms appear to occur more frequently in women. These findings raise questions as to whether BDD is a distinct diagnosis, because these symptoms occur in a large percentage of the population, especially women. These results, however, were obtained with the use of an apparently unvalidated questionnaire. In addition, while preoccupation with body image is widespread, this "normal" concern is clearly associated with less distress and impairment than is experienced by a clinical population with BDD who might present to plastic surgeons or psychiatrists. The proposed changes for DSM-IV reflect these differences with the addition of a new criterion for BDD: "The preoccupation causes significant impairment in social or occupational functioning, or causes marked distress (American Psychiatric Association 1991, p. I:8).

How do BDD patients differ from cosmetic surgery patients? An extensive literature exists dealing with psychological and psychiatric assessment in cosmetic surgery patients, although it is limited by a single-group, uncontrolled design and a lack of rigorous methodology for diagnosing BDD and other psychiatric disorders. Earlier psychiatric studies in cosmetic surgery applicants revealed a very high prevalence of psychiatric disorders in both female (53%–80%) and male (100%) candidates (Edgerton et al. 1961, 1964; Jacobson et al. 1960). However, later studies found lower rates (24%–32%) of psychiatric illness in surgical patients, which have been partially attributed to the greater acceptability of cosmetic surgery (Goin et al. 1980; Reich 1975; Shipley et al. 1977).

It is difficult to diagnose BDD among cosmetic surgery applicants. It is also difficult to predict which patients will have a poor response to cosmetic surgery, although patients with true dysmorphophobia (or BDD) have been hypothesized to differ from other cosmetic surgery patients by having more emotional problems, minimal objectively verified disfigurement, and poor surgical outcome with requests for additional operations (Turner et al. 1984). In one study, rhinoplasty patients with minimal objective disfigurement continued to request further surgery (Knorr et al. 1968). In a more recent study of BDD patients, a poor outcome following surgery was found (Phillips et al., in press). Unusual requests may in fact be a clue to the diagnosis of BDD and the possibility of poor outcome with surgery, but the prediction of surgical outcome may tax even an experienced psychiatrist.

Depersonalization Disorder

Similar diagnostic issues may be raised with DEP. Is DEP a discrete diagnostic entity? Does primary DEP differ from secondary DEP (i.e., a disorder that arises in the setting of another psychiatric illness)? What is the relationship between transient depersonalization symptoms and DEP?

Depersonalization disorder has been considered a discrete diagnostic entity, with an often sudden onset and chronic course. According to DSM-III-R, the diagnosis of DEP is not made when the symptom of depersonalization is secondary to any other disorder, such as panic disorder or agoraphobia without history of panic disorder. However, if depersonalization precedes or is independent of other disorders, it may be diagnosed as such. Nevertheless, the hierarchical exclusion of depersonalization in the presence of other disorders, particularly OCD and panic disorder, has been questioned (Hollander et al. 1990b). Further, there is little evidence that chronic DEP occurring in the setting of another disorder differs in a meaningful way from DEP occurring in isolation.

The symptom of depersonalization is quite common and has been experienced by 30% to 70% of young adult cohorts. Some studies suggest it is more common in young women; others do not find a gender difference (Kluft 1988). Depersonalization symptoms are also quite common in psychiatric populations. Up to 80% of hospitalized patients may have depersonalization symptoms, but these symptoms are severe or lasting in only 12% and are not the chief complaint (Brauer et al. 1970). The symptom of depersonalization may occur in association with schizophrenia, depression, phobic anxiety states, OCD, drug abuse, sleep deprivation, temporal lobe epilepsy, and migraine (Putnam 1985). Transient depersonalization symptoms are thus common in normal and psychiatric populations. However, in the vast majority of cases, these symptoms do not develop into depersonalization disorder.

Relationship to the Delusional Spectrum

Body Dysmorphic Disorder

The difference between BDD and DDST depends on whether the thoughts of a defect in appearance represent an overvalued idea (with uncertainty) as in the case of BDD (Thomas 1984), or reach delusional intensity (with certainty) as in the case of DDST, or monosymptomatic hypochondriacal psychosis (Munro and Chmara 1982). However, it has been unclear whether BDD and DDST are two different disorders (American Psychiatric Association 1987; Munro and Stewart 1991; Thomas 1985) or two variants of the same disorder (Brotman and Jenike 1985).

Hollander et al. (1989b) have suggested that patients with BDD can be placed along a continuum of insight or certainty. Patients at the extreme end who are currently classified as having DDST, or hypochondriacal psychosis, might be considered to have BDD with delusional features. Despite the possible existence of a phenomeno-logical spectrum, additional biological mechanisms may be involved in patients at the delusional end, with whom concerns become fixed beliefs.

Phillips et al. (in press) studied 30 patients with BDD and found that patients with delusional BDD symptoms did not differ from those with nondelusional symptoms in terms of demographic features, associated features or psychopathology, course of treatment, or treatment response. This finding suggests that the current division between BDD and DDST is largely arbitrary. Many BDD patients have a delusional conviction at various times in the course of their illness, and some have overvalued ideation with regard to one "defect" but delusional thinking with regard to another "defect." However, controlled studies in larger patient samples are needed prior to making major changes in our diagnostic classification systems, especially because the issue of delusional/nondelusional status has important implications for classification of other disorders as well, notably OCD and hypochondriasis.

This issue is addressed in the *DSM-IV Options Book* in the introduction to the section on BDD:

> There may [be] a continuum between the "preoccupation with an imagined defect" that is part of the definition of this disorder and the somatic delusions characteristic of Delusional Disorder, Somatic Type. A similar continuum between belief and delusion may also occur in Obsessive-Compulsive Disorder and Hypochondriasis. It has therefore been suggested that the proposed subtyping scheme for Obsessive-Compulsive Disorder (i.e., With Insight, With Overvalued Ideas, With Delusions) might be adopted for BDD. (American Psychiatric Association 1991, p. I:8)

Depersonalization Disorder

One change from the DSM-III (American Psychiatric Association 1980) to the DSM-III-R criteria for DEP was the addition of a criterion that the defect is not of delusional intensity (i.e., "during the depersonalization experience, reality testing remains intact") to minimize the possibility that early aspects of a psychotic experience could be misdiagnosed as DEP. Furthermore, depersonalization as a symptom of schizophrenia is specifically excluded in criterion D. Nevertheless, patients with DEP are often convinced that they are really experiencing their sensory misperceptions. This, in turn, raises the question of whether this disorder may in some cases be of delusional intensity.

Relationship to Obsessive-Compulsive Disorder

Phenomenology

Body dysmorphic disorder. Patients with BDD suffer from repetitive, persistent ideas or thoughts about their perceived body defects. However, some BDD patients do not experience intrusive or senseless ego-dystonic thoughts but rather ego-syntonic, overvalued beliefs. This is somewhat problematic for the argument that BDD and OCD are related, because OCD typically, but not always, is characterized by ego-dystonic obsessions.

However, this issue of ego-dystonic versus ego-syntonic obsessions may also relate to issues of uncertainty versus certainty. A review and phenomenological analysis of OCD by Insel and Akiskal (1986) suggested that delusions (ego-syntonic certainty) can arise in the course of this illness. These delusions do not signify a schizophrenic diagnosis but represent generally transient reactive affective or paranoid psychoses. The authors argued that OCD represents a psychopathological spectrum varying along a continuum of insight, with patients at the extreme end having an "obsessive compulsive psychosis" (Insel and Akiskal 1986). This spectrum has been described in depression (i.e., delusional depression) and social phobia (i.e., delusional belief of emitting a foul odor). A delusional spectrum has also been described, as noted above, for BDD in which ego-syntonic symptoms are viewed as realistic. Nevertheless, symptoms are "ego dystonic" in that these patients experience considerable dysphoria, anxiety, and functional impairment that bring them to the attention of clinicians.

A recent report has questioned the relationship between OCD and BDD based on the observation that BDD patients suffer from overvalued ideas rather than obsessions (Vitiello and DeLeon 1990). An overvalued idea was defined as a belief that is without objective justification and is not actively resisted. This belief was said to differ from a delusion, which was defined as fixed and unshakeable, and from an obsession, which was defined as ego-dystonic, intrusive, and one that is resisted. However, as described above, certainty of belief may exist on a continuum in both BDD and OCD, and patients may at different stages of their illness have true obsessions, overvalued ideas, or delusions.

Some authors have suggested that "obsessive-compulsiveness" (Hollander et al. 1989b; Hunecke and Bosse 1985) or obsessive or compulsive personality traits (Andreason and Bardach 1977; Hollander et al. 1989b; Hunecke and Bosse 1985; Thomas 1984) are a hallmark of BDD. However, other diagnoses such as depression with ruminations or generalized anxiety disorder may also have obsessional features. Further, obsessive-compulsive personality disorder (OCPD) and traits differ from those of OCD. Most patients with OCD do not have coexistent OCPD; in addition, most patients with OCPD do not develop OCD (Rasmussen and Tsuang 1986). Nevertheless, these case reports suggest a high rate of obsessive-compulsive symptoms and personality traits in patients with BDD (Hollander et al. 1989b; Phillips et al., in press).

Depersonalization disorder.   Both OCD and DEP involve repetitive ego-dystonic thoughts. In OCD, these disturbing thoughts usually focus on uncertainty and are characterized by an exaggerated perception of future harm. In DEP, they center on discomfort and sensory perceptual distortions involving the self or body and its relation to the world.

Previous studies have posited a link between obsessional personality traits and depersonalization (Torch 1978). Two series reported an 88% and 75% incidence of premorbid obsessional traits in depersonalized patients (Roth 1959; Torch 1978, respectively). Torch (1978) initially distinguished between two variants of depersonalization: 1) an intellectual-obsessive depersonalization characterized by alternating states of depersonalization and morbid self-scrutiny, which is found primarily in males who have highly obsessive premorbid personalities; and 2) a form of depression characterized more by prominent feelings of derealization, which occurs more commonly in women.

Torch (1981) postulated that depersonalization involves an obsessional repetition of an initial experience of unreality. He noted an undeniable presence of both obsessional personality characteristics and an OCD-like tendency toward a continuous and compulsive reliving of the state. This work was partly based on the work of Skoog (1965), who noted that in the onset of anancastic conditions, depersonalization and obsession merge with each another phenomenologically. The patient is obsessionally driven to get to the bottom of his or her agonizing experience and experiences both alienation and a reinforced feeling of unreality.

Roth's (1959) concept of the phobic anxiety–depersonalization syndrome included patients who might now be diagnosed with Briquet's syndrome, conversion hysteria, or hysterical personality; these patients also suffered from fleeting and transient depersonalization and obsessional patterns of thought and behavior. However, they were found to respond to the standard tricyclic antidepressant imipramine (Klein 1964), whereas patients with DEP generally do not respond to this agent (Hollander et al. 1989a). This finding suggests that the phobic anxiety depersonalization syndrome may differ in some respects from DEP.

In another study, three of eight patients with DEP had obsessions and/or compulsions (Hollander et al. 1990b). These patients, in whom the presence of obsessional symptoms or OCD was a good prognostic sign, had the most favorable response to serotonin (5-hydroxytryptamine [5-HT]) reuptake blockers. They experienced at least partial resolution of obsessional symptoms as well.

Course of Illness

Body dysmorphic disorder. Although there are no systematic follow-up studies of BDD, this disorder appears to be a chronic illness that, if not successfully treated, remains stable for many years, if not decades (Frances and Oldham 1986; Hollander et al. 1989b; Phillips et al., in press). Related syndromes such as olfactory reference syndrome (a form of monosymptomatic hypochondriasis) and monosymptomatic psychogenic eye pain also have a chronic course with poor prognosis (Bebbington 1976; Bishop 1980). Cosmetic surgery reports of patients with probable BDD suggest that over the long term, cosmetic operations often do not change the patients' perceptions of their so-called deformations (Connolly and Gipson 1978;

Kuchenhoff 1984), and these reports imply that the course of BDD is often chronic.

Depersonalization disorder. There are no large-scale follow-up studies of DEP, and thus information is limited to anecdotal case reports. The onset of DEP is usually rapid, and its disappearance is usually gradual (American Psychiatric Association 1987). Even with treatment, the course is generally chronic, with remissions and exacerbations (Kluft 1988). Psychosocial stress may be followed by symptom exacerbation, and comorbid Axis II illness may worsen the long-term outcome.

Obsessive-compulsive disorder Follow-up studies of OCD are limited, but one study reported that the course of OCD could be divided into three categories: 1) unremitting and chronic, 2) phasic with periods of complete remission, and 3) episodic with incomplete remissions (Goodwin et al. 1969). According to DSM-III-R, the course is usually chronic, with waxing and waning symptoms. Comorbid cluster A (odd) or cluster B (impulsive) personality disorders have been associated with a poorer outcome (Baer et al., unpublished data, 1992).

Thus all three disorders appear to have a chronic course, although prospective follow-up studies are needed.

Prevalence

Body dysmorphic disorder. The prevalence of BDD is unknown, but because patients with this disorder are secretive and often present to plastic surgeons or dermatologists rather than psychiatrists, its prevalence may be much greater than is generally realized. It has been estimated that 2% of patients requesting cosmetic surgery may have BDD (Andreason and Bardach 1977; Fukuda 1977). Estimates of dysmorphophobic somatic delusions (body dysmorphic psychosis) range from 0.4% to 10% (Refsum et al. 1983; Retterstøl 1968; Winokur 1977). It is not known whether nonpsychotic forms of BDD are more or less common than body dysmorphic psychosis.

Depersonalization disorder. The prevalence of DEP is also unknown. The symptom of depersonalization is quite common and has been experienced in up to 70% of young adult cohorts (Kluft 1988) and 80% of psychiatric patients (Brauer et al. 1970). However, these subjects did not have the severity, distress, interference with functioning, or chronicity associated with DEP.

Obsessive-compulsive disorder. Recent estimates of the lifetime prevalence of OCD suggest a rate of 2% to 3% in the general population, although this rate probably includes subclinical cases (Robins et al. 1984).

While obsessive-compulsive, dysmorphophobic, and depersonalization symptoms are very common, true OCD appears more common than either BDD or DEP. However, the latter two disorders may be underdiagnosed, and studies of BDD and DEP similar to that of the Epidemiologic Catchment Area study are needed.

Age at Onset

Body dysmorphic disorder. Most cases in the literature suggest that BDD begins in early adolescence through the 20s (Andreason and Bardach 1977; Hollander et al. 1989b; Kuchenhoff 1984; Phillips et al., in press; Thomas 1984). However, BDD may not be diagnosed for years after its onset because patients may be reluctant to reveal their symptoms, which they often consider embarrassing and humiliating (Andreason and Bardach 1977; Phillips et al., in press).

Depersonalization disorder. Depersonalization disorder usually begins in adolescence or early adulthood, with onset rarely after age 40. The onset of DEP has been noted to sometimes be precipitated by panic attacks, marijuana, or caffeine.

Obsessive-compulsive disorder. Obsessive-compulsive disorder has a reported mean age at onset of 20 years, with 65% of patients developing their illness prior to age 25 (Rasmussen and Tsuang 1986). Like BDD, OCD may not be diagnosed for years after its onset.

Thus all three disorders have an early age at onset—most commonly adolescence or early adulthood.

Comorbidity and Impairment

Body dysmorphic disorder. There is a high rate of comorbid affective, anxiety, and personality disorder diagnoses in BDD (Andreason and Bardach 1977; Connolly and Gipson 1978; Frances and Oldham 1986; Hollander et al. 1989b; Phillips et al., in press; Signer and Benson 1987; Sturmey and Slade 1986; Thomas 1984). In addition, BDD has been reported to have a fairly high comorbidity with OCD (E. Hollander, unpublished observations; Phillips et al., in press). In terms of predisposing and comorbid personality traits, BDD patients are often perfectionistic and may have obsessional, compulsive, schizoid, or narcissistic traits (Andreason and Bardach 1977; Thomas 1984). However, personality traits have not been assessed in these patients in a systematic fashion.

Social and occupational functioning may be severely impaired in BDD patients, and this impairment may be exacerbated by prolonged searches for surgical or dermatological cure.

Depersonalization disorder. Depersonalization is often reported to occur in association with other syndromes, such as depression (Tucker et al. 1973), schizophrenia (Davison 1964; Tucker et al. 1973), temporal lobe epilepsy and complex partial seizures (Davison 1964; Greenberg et al. 1984), anxiety disorders (Nuller 1982) and phobic anxiety–depersonalization syndrome (Roth 1959), migraines (Comfort 1982), marijuana abuse (Szymanski 1981), and even in some analogue and "normal" student populations (Myers and Grant 1972). While the symptom of depersonalization is encountered with these other symptoms, the disorder, DEP, is diagnosed only if the symptom is persistent or recurrent, and causes distress.

In a study of eight patients with depersonalization, seven had associated panic or obsessive-compulsive symptoms; two of these patients had depersonalization symptoms secondary to OCD or panic disorder, and thus the diagnosis of DEP was hierarchically excluded (Hollander et al. 1990b). Six patients had depersonalization symptoms that preceded or were independent of associated disorders, or did not have associated disorders, and thus met the DSM-III-R criteria for DEP.

Obsessive-compulsive disorder. Like BDD and DEP, OCD has a high rate of comorbid affective, anxiety, and personality disorder diagnoses (Rasmussen and Tsuang 1986), and it is often associated with severe impairment in social and occupational functioning.

Treatment

Body dysmorphic disorder. Treatment studies of BDD are limited to anecdotal case reports or small open clinical trials. Isolated case reports have described improvement in dysmorphophobia following treatment with psychoanalytically oriented psychotherapy (Bloch and Glue 1988; Philippopoulos 1979). There have also been reports of successful behavioral treatment of dysmorphophobia with systematic desensitization (Munjack 1978) and systematic exposure to avoided situations that evoke dysmorphophobic discomfort (Marks and Mishan 1988), a behavioral approach that is also a highly effective treatment for OCD. Other investigators suggest the usefulness of a cognitive-behavioral approach that is the reverse of that used for anorexic patients (Jerome 1987). Photodrama, the discovery of new aspects of the self through photographs, has been used to treat adolescents and young adults with body-image problems (Castro et al. 1973; Ehrlich and Tomkiewicz 1980).

Several case reports have documented some improvement in the delusional version of BDD (monosymptomatic hypochondriasis) and in nondelusional BDD with tricyclic antidepressants (Brotman and Jenike 1984; Fernando 1988) and MAO inhibitors (Jenike 1984). However, a larger number of reports document an unsuccessful outcome with these medications (Braddock 1982; Campanella 1968; Cotterill 1981; Hollander et al. 1989b; Phillips et al., in press). Improvement in monosymptomatic hypochondriacal psychosis and monosymptomatic parisitophobia (i.e., fear of lice infestation) has also been reported with pimozide (Munro and Chmara 1982; Rapp 1986; Riding and Munro 1975).

Hollander et al. (1989b) reported on five patients with body dysmorphic symptoms that were previously refractory to a variety of somatic treatments. These patients substantially improved following open treatment with the serotonin reuptake blockers clomipramine and/or fluoxetine, suggesting that there was a selective 5-HT effect. Phillips et al. (in press) have also reported a preferential response to serotonin reuptake blockers in 30 patients with BDD. Because these agents have selective antiobsessional effects in OCD (DeVeaugh-Geiss et al. 1989; Liebowitz et al. 1989; Thorén et al. 1980a), these findings raise the possibility of a common pathogenesis with OCD, although they do not exclude a possible antidepressant effect or a relationship of BDD with affective illness. However, standard antidepressants and ECT are usually ineffective in BDD, suggesting that the anti-BDD effect of serotonin reuptake blockers is not merely an antidepressant effect. In addition, Phillips et al. (in press) found that the rate of response to serotonergic antidepressants did not differ significantly in patients with or without comorbid major depression.

A recent case report described one patient with dysmorphophobia who failed to respond to clomipramine (200 mg/day) (Vitiello and DeLeon 1990). However, even in OCD, only 60% of patients respond to a trial of a single serotonin reuptake blocker (DeVeaugh-Geiss et al. 1989), necessitating augmentation strategies or a switch to another 5-HT agent.

Depersonalization disorder. Previous case reports have documented improvement of depersonalization symptoms with antidepressants (Klein 1964; Walsh 1975), stimulants (Cattell 1966; Davison 1964), benzodiazepines (Greenberg et al. 1984), barbiturates (King and Little 1959), and antiepileptics (Greenberg et al. 1984). Hypnosis, behavior modification, family therapy, ECT, and prefrontal leukotomy have also been reported to be effective in individual cases.

One open study found preferential response of depersonalization symptoms or DEP to agents that manifest potent serotonin reuptake blockade (Hollander et al. 1990b). Chronic depersonalization symptoms resolved in six of eight patients treated with fluoxetine or fluvoxamine. Not all patients with DEP responded to all serotonin reuptake blockers; one patient did not improve with clomipramine but did respond to fluvoxamine. One patient with evidence of cerebral dysrhythmia on the EEG and one patient with no history of panic or obsessive-compulsive symptoms failed to improve with fluoxetine.

The chronicity of DEP, coupled with a poor response to prior somatic and psychological treatments, makes the positive therapeutic response of depersonalization to 5-HT reuptake blockers noteworthy. Further work is needed to clarify whether patients with DEP and coexistent OCD or panic disorder are particularly responsive to treatment with these agents.

Presumed Etiology

Serotonergic models

In Chapter 1, it was noted that a subgroup of patients with OCD may manifest an abnormality of central serotonergic function based on studies of pharmacological response (DeVeaugh-Geiss et al. 1989; Liebowitz et al. 1989; Thorén et al. 1980a), cerebrospinal fluid 5-hydroxyindoleacetic acid (5-HIAA) (Thorén et al. 1980b), and peripheral platelet imipramine binding (Flament et al. 1987). Furthermore, administration of oral m-chlorophenylpiperazine (m-CPP), a selective 5-HT agonist, has been shown to exacerbate OCD symptoms transiently (Hollander et al. 1988, 1992; Zohar et al. 1987), and chronic clomipramine (Zohar et al. 1988) or fluoxetine (Hollander et al. 1991a) treatment has been shown to reverse behavioral and neuro-endocrine abnormalities in OCD.

Body dysmorphic disorder. Patients with BDD seem to respond preferentially to serotonin reuptake blockers, which is consistent with the possibility of serotonergic dysregulation in some BDD patients. There have been reports of exacerbation of body dysmorphic symptoms of delusional intensity with smoking of marijuana (Hollander et al. 1989b), which has central 5-HT effects. However, this is not a selective 5-HT–provocative test, because marijuana affects several other neurotransmitter systems, including acetylcholine. A fascinating case report of a woman who developed BDD following chronic abuse of cyproheptadine, a serotonin antagonist, does make the possibility of a serotonergic etiology intriguing (Craven and Rodin 1987).

Depersonalization disorder. Selective response of some cases of DEP to 5-HT reuptake blockers (Hollander et al. 1990b), co-occurrence with migraines (Comfort 1982), exacerbation by marijuana (Szymanski 1981), and overlap with OCD and panic disorder (Hollander et al. 1990b) all indirectly implicate serotonergic involvement in DEP, although other neurotransmitter systems may also have some role.

Neurological models

An alternative hypothesis regarding OCD involves organic disturbance in a subgroup of OCD patients. In particular, there are reports of the onset of OCD following von Economo's disease (Schilder 1938) as well as other types of encephalitis and meningitis (Grimshaw 1964). A subgroup of OCD patients have increased neurological soft signs (Behar et al. 1984; Bihari et al. 1991; Hollander et al. 1990c), neuropsychological and visuospatial abnormalities (Behar et al. 1984; Hollander et al. 1991b), and abnormalities on computed tomography (Behar et al. 1984; Luxenberg et al. 1988) and positron-emission tomography scans (Baxter et al. 1987; Swedo et al. 1989), suggesting a neurological etiology in some patients with this disorder.

Body dysmorphic disorder. There are reports of BDD occurring following infection in children (Carek and Santos 1984) and subacute sclerosing panencephalitis in early adulthood (Salib 1988).

Depersonalization disorder. In DEP, case reports document an association with temporal lobe epilepsy and complex partial seizures (Davison 1964; Greenberg et al. 1984) and migraines (Comfort 1982). There are also documented abnormalities in EEG (Hollander et al. 1990b), SPECT, neurometrics, and neurological soft signs in some DEP patients that are reflective of findings in OCD (see Case 2 presented earlier in this chapter).

Relationship of Obsessive-Compulsive Disorder, Body Dysmorphic Disorder, and Depersonalization Disorder to Other Disorders

Anorexia Nervosa

Patients with anorexia nervosa frequently have obsessive-compulsive symptoms (Gomez and Dally 1980; Hollander 1991; Morgan and Russell 1975), and OCD patients have high rates of anorexia nervosa by history (Kasvikis et al. 1986; Rasmussen and Eisen 1988; Solyom et al. 1982).

Anorexic persons avoid mirrors and perceive themselves as being fatter than they are, whereas dysmorphophobic individuals either excessively check or else avoid mirrors and perceive a defect in one particular aspect of their appearance rather than their body weight (Apfelbaum et al. 1973; Jerome 1987; Thomas 1987). However, some anorexic individuals also focus on one aspect of their appearance that to them seems overweight, such as their calves. Although it has been suggested that opposite cognitive-behavioral approaches may be used for anorexic and dysmorphophobic patients, with mirror confrontation for the former and mirror avoidance for the latter (Jerome 1987), the usefulness of these strategies requires further empirical support.

Social Phobia

Body dysmorphic disorder may also be related to social phobia, because both disorders are characterized by an excessive fear of negative social evaluation. BDD is in fact classified as a type of social phobia in Japan, and Marks (1980) actually defined dysmorphophobia as a type of social phobia, evidenced by high anxiety in social situations, avoidance of such situations, and fear of criticism. BDD and social phobia both have an early age at onset, and case reports of BDD highlight associated shyness and avoidant features (Braddock 1982; Olley 1974; Phillips et al., in press; Sturmey and Slade 1986).

Panic

Depersonalization frequently occurs in the setting of a panic attack. The phobic anxiety–depersonalization syndrome described by Roth (1959) featured depersonalization symptoms associated with panic anxiety. In one study (Hollander et al. 1990b), four of five patients with DEP who had previous or current histories of panic attacks improved markedly with serotonin reuptake blockers, which also have antipanic effects (Sheehan et al. 1988). This antidepersonalization response was not simply an antipanic response, since other antipanic medications, including imipramine, alprazolam, and diazepam, successfully treated the panic attacks but did not affect depersonalization symptoms (Hollander et al. 1989a).

Depressive Disorders

Depression has been reported to be the most common comorbid illness in OCD (Rasmussen and Tsuang 1986), DEP (Brauer et al. 1970; Davison 1964; Roth 1959; Sedman 1972; Sedman and Reed 1963; Shorvon 1946; Skoog 1965) and BDD (Cotterill 1981; de Leon et al. 1989; Hardy 1982; Hay 1970; Hollander et al. 1989b; Marks and Mishan 1988; Phillips et al., in press; Thomas 1984). While there appears to be an elevated rate of mood disorder in the families of BDD patients (Andreason and Bardach 1977; Hay 1970; Hollander et al. 1989b; Jenike 1984; Phillips et al., in press), this could also reflect an increased rate of depression in the probands.

However, the link between OCD, DEP, or BDD, and affective disorders is weakened by the poor response of OCD, DEP, and BDD to ECT (Hay 1970; Hollander et al. 1989b; Phillips et al., in press; Thomas 1985) and to typical antidepressants (Hollander et al. 1990b; Phillips 1991).

Summary

Body dysmorphic disorder shares many similarities with OCD, as well as with some cases of cosmetic surgery, anorexia nervosa, social phobia, and depression. However, most of the existing evidence stems from anecdotal case reports, and there remains a paucity of large systematic studies of BDD. There is little evidence linking BDD to other somatoform disorders; furthermore, as individual patients progress through the course of their illness, their diagnosis may shift from a somatoform to a delusional disorder or vice versa, suggesting problems with the DSM-III-R differentiation of BDD and its delusional variant. Large systematic studies of BDD are needed. The DSM-IV field trial of OCD will assess BDD symptoms in a large number of OCD patients at five sites and will compare findings in the OCD population with those in a BDD sample. This trial may generate much needed data about the relationship between BDD and OCD, and may inform diagnostic considerations in DSM-IV and beyond.

Depersonalization disorder may also share many similarities with OCD, including phenomenology, course of illness, age at onset, comorbidity, treatment response, and serotonergic and neuropsychiatric findings. Many DEP patients have premorbid obsessional traits. However, there are also differences between the two disorders, and DEP may occur in the setting of several disorders. Co-occurrence of obsessive-compulsive or panic symptoms in DEP patients has been associated with a favorable response of depersonalization symptoms to serotonin reuptake blockers.

Conclusions

In this chapter we have reviewed diagnostic issues in BDD and DEP and discussed the relationship of these disorders to OCD and other disorders. The lack of systematic studies of BDD and DEP makes it difficult to assess the validity of these disorders as subgroups of OCD, or even as distinct diagnostic entities. Controversy focuses on whether these disorders are primary or secondary and to what extent they overlap with normal populations. The current diagnostic system for BDD creates additional difficulties because there is an overlap with delusional disorder, somatic type (monosymptomatic delusional hypochondriasis). Patients may be classified as having a somatoform disorder at one stage of their illness and a delusional disorder at another stage of the same illness, raising the question of whether these disorders are actually the same.

Despite the limitations of the available data and the need for controlled studies, external validators, such as age at onset, clinical course, comorbidity, impairment, prevalence, treatment implications, and possible etiologies, suggest that BDD and DEP may be related to OCD. It is of potential clinical importance to assess obsessive-compulsive symptoms in patients with BDD and DEP and to look for body dysmorphic and depersonalization symptoms in patients with OCD. Behavioral techniques (i.e., exposure and response prevention) and medications (i.e., clomipramine, fluoxetine, fluvoxamine) that have documented efficacy in OCD may prove useful in BDD and DEP. It remains to be determined whether BDD and DEP patients with symptoms of OCD have a better response to antiobsessional treatments than do those patients without OCD symptoms. Further, it is not known whether OCD patients with BDD or DEP symptoms have a worse prognosis than do those without these symptoms. Finally, appreciating that BDD and DEP may lie within a spectrum of OCD/OCD-related disorders may enhance communication between researchers studying these various disorders.

References

American Psychiatric Association: Diagnostic and Statistical Manual of Mental Disorders, 3rd Edition. Washington, DC, American Psychiatric Association, 1980

American Psychiatric Association: Diagnostic and Statistical Manual of Mental Disorders, 3rd Edition, Revised. Washington, DC, American Psychiatric Association, 1987

American Psychiatric Association: DSM-IV Options Book: Work In Progress (9/1/91). Washington DC, American Psychiatric Association, 1991

Andreasen NC, Bardach J: Dysmorphophobia: symptom or disease? Am J Psychiatry 134:673–676, 1977

Apfelbaum M, Igoin L: Obesity, bulimia, and dysmorphophobia. Revue de Medecine Psychosomatique et de Psychologie Medicale 15:125–130, 1973

Baxter LR Jr, Phelps ME, Mazziotta JC, et al: Local cerebral glucose metabolic rates in obsessive-compulsive disorder: a comparison with rates in unipolar depression and in normal controls. Arch Gen Psychiatry 44:211–218, 1987

Bebbington PE: Monosymptomatic hypochondriasis, abnormal illness behaviour and suicide. Br J Psychiatry 128:475–478, 1976

Behar D, Rapoport JL, Berg CJ, et al: Computerized tomography and neuropsychological test measures in adolescents with obsessive-compulsive disorder. Am J Psychiatry 141:363–369, 1984

Bihari K, Pato MT, Hill JL, et al: Neurological soft signs in obsessive-compulsive disorder (letter). Arch Gen Psychiatry 48:278, 1991

Bishop ER: An olfactory reference syndrome—monosymptomatic hypochondriasis. J Clin Psychiatry 41:57–59, 1980

Bloch S, Glue P: Psychotherapy and dysmorphophobia: a case report. Br J Psychiatry 152:271–274, 1988

Braddock LE: Dysmorphophobia in adolescence: a case report. Br J Psychiatry 140:199–201, 1982

Brauer R, Harrow M, Tucker GJ: Depersonalization phenomena in psychiatric patients. Br J Psychiatry 117:509–515, 1970

Brotman AW, Jenike MA: Monosymptomatic hypochondriasis treated with tricyclic antidepressants. Am J Psychiatry 141:1608–1609, 1984

Brotman AW, Jenike MA: Dysmorphophobia and monosymptomatic hypochondriasis (reply to letter by Thomas CS). Am J Psychiatry 142:1121, 1985

Campanella FN, Zuccoli E: In tema di dismorfobia. Neuropsichiatria 24:475–486, 1968

Carek DJ, Santos AB Jr: Atypical somatoform disorder following infection in children: a depressive equivalent? J Clin Psychiatry 45:108–111, 1984

Castro L, Finder J, Tomkiewicz S: Dysmorphophobia in the young girl and its treatment through photodrama. Bulletin de Psychologie 27:117–127, 1973

Catell JP: Depersonalization phenomena, in American Handbook of Psychiatry, Vol 3. Edited by Arieti S. New York, Basic Books, 1966, pp 88–100

Comfort A: Out-of-body experiences and migraine (letter). Am J Psychiatry 139:1379–1380, 1982

Connolly FH, Gipson M: Dysmorphophobia—a long-term study. Br J Psychiatry 132:568–570, 1978

Cotterill JA: Dermatologic non-disease: a common and potentially fatal disturbance of cutaneous body image. Br J Dermatol 104:611–619, 1981

Craven JL, Rodin GM: Cyproheptadine dependence associated with an atypical somatoform disorder. Can J Psychiatry 32:143–145, 1987

Davison K: Episodic depersonalization: observations on 7 patients. Br J Psychiatry 110:505–513, 1964

DeVeaugh-Geiss J, Landau P, Katz R: Treatment of obsessive compulsive disorder with clomipramine. Psychiatric Annals 19:97–101, 1989

de Leon J, Bott A, Simpson GM: Dysmorphophobia: body dysmorphic disorder or delusional disorder, somatic subtype? Compr Psychiatry 30:457–472, 1989

Edgerton MT, Meyer E, Jacobson WE: Augmentation mammoplasty, II: further surgical and psychiatric evaluation. Plast Reconstr Surg 27:279–302, 1961

Edgerton MT, Webb WL, Slaughter R, et al: Surgical results and psychosocial changes following rhytidectomy: an evaluation of face lifting. Plast Reconstr Surg 33:503–521, 1964

Ehrlich P, Tomkiewicz S: Le photodrame: apprentissage et transmissibilité. Bulletin de Psychologie 34:853–860, 1980

Fernando N: Monosymptomatic hypochondriasis treated with a tricyclic antidepressant. Br J Psychiatry 152:851–852, 1988

Fitts SN, Gibson P, Redding CA, et al: Body dysmorphic disorder: implications for its validity as a DSM-III-R clinical syndrome. Psychol Rep 64:655–658, 1989

Flament MF, Rapoport JL, Murphy DL, et al: Biochemical changes during clomipramine treatment of childhood obsessive-compulsive disorder. Arch Gen Psychiatry 44:219–225, 1987

Frances A, Oldham J: Unsuccessful treatment of a 45-year-old man with delusions of somatic disorders. Hosp Community Psychiatry 37:993–994, 1986

Fukuda O: Statistical analysis of dysmorphophobia in out-patient clinic. Japanese Journal of Plastic and Reconstructive Surgery 20:569–577, 1977

Goin MK, Burgoyne RW, Goin JM, et al: A prospective psychological study of 50 female face-lift patients. Plast Reconstr Surg 65:436–442, 1980

Gomez J, Dally P: Psychometric rating in assessment of progress in anorexia nervosa. Br J Psychiatry 136:290–296, 1980

Goodwin DW, Guze SB, Robins E: Follow-up studies in obsessional neurosis. Arch Gen Psychiatry 20:182–187, 1969

Greenberg DB, Hochberg FH, Murray GB: The theme of death in complex partial seizures. Am J Psychiatry 141:1587–1589, 1984

Grimshaw L: Obsessional disorder and neurological illness. J Neurol Neurosurg Psychiatry 27:229–231, 1964

Hardy GE: Body image disturbance in dysmorphophobia. Br J Psychiatry 141:181–185, 1982

Hay GG: Dysmorphophobia. Br J Psychiatry 116:399–406, 1970

Hollander E: Serotonergic drugs and the treatment of disorders related to obsessive-compulsive disorder, in Current Treatments of Obsessive-Compulsive Disorder. Edited by Pato MT, Zohar J. Washington, DC, American Psychiatric Press, 1991, pp 173–191

Hollander E, Fay M, Cohen B, et al: Serotonergic and noradrenergic sensitivity in obsessive-compulsive disorder: behavioral findings. Am J Psychiatry 145:1015–1017, 1988

Hollander E, Fairbanks J, DeCaria C, et al: Pharmacological dissection of panic and depersonalization (letter). Am J Psychiatry 146:402, 1989a

Hollander E, Liebowitz MR, Winchel R, et al: Treatment of body-dysmorphic disorder with serotonin reuptake blockers. Am J Psychiatry 146:768–770, 1989b

Hollander E, DeCaria C, Liebowitz MR, et al: Body dysmorphic disorder (letter reply to Thomas CS). Am J Psychiatry 147:817, 1990a

Hollander E, Liebowitz MR, DeCaria C, et al: Treatment of depersonalization with serotonin reuptake blockers. J Clin Psychopharmacol 10:200–203, 1990b

Hollander E, Schiffman E, Cohen B, et al: Signs of central nervous system dysfunction in obsessive-compulsive disorder. Arch Gen Psychiatry 47:27–32, 1990c

Hollander E, DeCaria C, Gully R, et al: Effects of chronic fluoxetine treatment on behavioral and neuroendocrine responses to meta-chloro-phenylpiperazine in obsessive-compulsive disorder. Psychiatry Res 36:1–17, 1991a

Hollander E, Liebowitz MR, Rosen W: Neuropsychiatric and neuropsychological function in obsessive-compulsive disorder, in The Psychobiology of Obsessive-Compulsive Disorder. Edited by Zohar J, Insel T, Rasmussen S. New York, Springer, 1991b, pp 126–145

Hollander E, DeCaria CM, Nitescu A, et al: Serotonergic function in obsessive-compulsive disorder: behavioral and neuroendocrine responses to oral m-chlorophenylpiperazine and fenfluramine in patients and healthy volunteers. Arch Gen Psychiatry 49:21–28, 1992

Hunecke P, Bosse K: Dysmorphophobia as casus pro diagnosi. Z Hautkr 60:1986–1989, 1985

Insel TR, Akiskal HS: Obsessive-compulsive disorder with psychotic features: a phenomenologic analysis. Am J Psychiatry 143:1527–1533, 1986

Jacobson WE, Edgerton MT, Meyer E, et al: Psychiatric evaluation of male patients seeking cosmetic surgery. Plast Reconstr Surg 26:356–372, 1960

Jenike MA: A case report of successful treatment of dysmorphophobia with tranylcypromine. Am J Psychiatry 141:1463–1464, 1984

Jerome L: Anorexia nervosa or dysmorphophobia (letter)? Br J Psychiatry 150:560–561, 1987

Kasvikis YG, Tsakiris F, Marks IM, et al: Past history of anorexia nervosa in women with obsessive-compulsive disorder. International Journal of Eating Disorders 5:1069–1075, 1986

King A, Little JC: Thiopentane treatment of the phobic anxiety depersonalization syndrome. Proc R Soc Med 52:595–596, 1959

Klein DF: Delineation of two drug-responsive anxiety syndromes. Psychopharmacology (Berlin) 5:397–408, 1964

Kluft RP: The dissociative disorders, in The American Psychiatric Press Textbook of Psychiatry. Edited by Talbott JA, Hales RE, Yudofsky SC. Washington, DC. American Psychiatric Press, 1988, pp 557–585

Knorr NJ, Hoopes JE, Edgerton MT: Psychiatric surgical approach to adolescent disturbance in self-image. Plast Reconstr Surg 41:248–253, 1968

Kuchenhoff J: Dysmorphophobia. Nervenarzt 55:122–123, 1984

Liebowitz MR, Hollander E, Schneier F, et al: Fluoxetine treatment of obsessive-compulsive disorder: an open clinical trial. J Clin Psychopharmacol 9:423–427, 1989

Luxenberg JS, Swedo SE, Flament MF, et al: Neuroanatomical abnormalities in obsessive-compulsive disorder detected with quantitative X-ray computed tomography. Am J Psychiatry 145:1089–1093, 1988

Marks IM: Cure and Care of Neurosis: Theory and Practice of Behavioral Psychotherapy. New York, Wiley, 1980

Marks IM, Mishan J: Dysmorphophobic avoidance with disturbed bodily perception: a pilot study of exposure therapy. Br J Psychiatry 152:674–678, 1988

Morgan HG, Russell GFM: Value of family background and clinical features as predictors of long-term outcome in anorexia nervosa: four-year follow-up study of 41 patients. Psychol Med 5:355–371, 1975

Munjack DJ: The behavioral treatment of dysmorphophobia. J Behav Ther Exp Psychiatry 9:53–56, 1978

Munro A, Chmara J: Monosymptomatic hypochondriacal psychosis: a diagnostic checklist based on 50 cases of the disorder. Can J Psychiatry 27:374–376, 1982

Munro A, Stewart M: Body dysmorphic disorder and the DSM-IV: the demise of dysmorphophobia. Can J Psychiatry 36:91–96, 1991

Myers DH, Grant G: A study of depersonalization in students. Br J Psychiatry 121:59–65, 1972

Nuller YL. Depersonalization—symptoms, meaning, therapy. Acta Psychiatr. Scand 66:451–458, 1982

Olley PC: Psychiatric aspects of referral (in Aspects of Plastic Surgery column). BMJ 3:248–249, 1974

Philippopoulos GS: The analysis of a case of dysmorphophobia (psychopathology and psychodynamics). Can J Psychiatry 24:397–401, 1979

Phillips KA: Body dysmorphic disorder: the distress of imagined ugliness. Am J Psychiatry 148:1138–1149, 1991

Phillips KA, Hollander E: Body dysmorphic disorder, in DSM-IV Source Book. Edited by Widiger T. Washington, DC, American Psychiatric Press (in press)

Phillips KA, McElroy SL, Keck PE Jr, et al: Body dysmorphic disorder: 30 cases of imagined ugliness. Am J Psychiatry (in press)

Putnam FW Jr: Dissociation as a response to extreme trauma, in Childhood Antecedents of Multiple Personality. Edited by Kluft RP. Washington, DC, American Psychiatric Press, 1985, pp 65–97

Rapp MS: Monosymptomatic hypochondriasis (letter). Can J Psychiatry 31:599, 1986

Rasmussen SA, Eisen JL: Clinical and epidemiologic findings of significance to neuropharmacologic trials in OCD. Psychopharmacol Bull 24:466–470, 1988

Rasmussen SA, Tsuang MT: Clinical characteristics and family history in DSM-III obsessive-compulsive disorder. Am J Psychiatry 143:317–322, 1986

Refsum HE, Zivanovic S, Astrup C: Paranoiac psychoses: a follow-up. Neuropsychobiology 10:75–82, 1983

Reich J: Factors influencing patient satisfaction with the results of esthetic plastic surgery. Plast Reconstr Surg 55:5–13, 1975

Retterstol N: Paranoid psychoses with hypochondriac delusions as the main delusion: a personal follow-up investigation. Acta Psychiatr Scand 44:334–353, 1968

Riding J, Munro A: Pimozide in the treatment of monosymptomatic hypochondriacal psychosis. Acta Psychiatr Scand 52:23–30, 1975

Robins LN, Helzer JE, Weissman MM, et al: Lifetime prevalence of specific psychiatric disorders in three sites. Arch Gen Psychiatry 41:949–958, 1984

Roth M: The phobic anxiety depersonalization syndrome. Journal of Neuropsychiatry 1:293–306, 1959

Salib EA: Subacute sclerosing panencephalitis (SSPE) presenting at the age of 21 as a schizophrenia-like state with bizarre dysmorphophobic features. Br J Psychiatry 152:709–710, 1988

Schilder P: The organic background of obsessions and compulsions. Am J Psychiatry 94:1397–1416, 1938

Sedman G: An investigation of certain factors concerneed in the etiology of depersonalization. Acta Psychiatr Scand 48:191–219, 1972

Sedman G, Reed G: Depersonalization phenomena in obsessional personalities and in depression. Br J Psychiatry 109:669–673, 1963

Sheehan DV, Zak JP, Miller JA Jr, et al: Panic disorder: the potential role of serotonin reuptake inhibitors. J Clin Psychiatry 49 (no 8, suppl):30–36, 1988

Shipley RH, O'Donnell JM, Bader KF: Personality characteristics of women seeking breast augmentation. Plast Reconstr Surg 60:369–376, 1977

Shorvon H: The depersonalization syndrome. Proceedings of the Royal Society of Medicine 39:779–792, 1946

Signer SF, Benson DF: Two cases of Capgras symptom with dysmorphic (somatic) delusions. Psychosomatics 28:327–328, 1987

Skoog G: Onset of anancastic conditions. Acta Psychiatr Scand Suppl 184:67–78, 1965

Solyom L, Freeman RJ, Miles JE: A comparative psychometric study of anorexia nervosa and obsessive neurosis. Can J Psychiatry 27:282–286, 1982

Sturmey P, Slade PD: Anorexia nervosa and dysmorphophobia: a case study. Br J Psychiatry 149:780–782, 1986

Swedo SE, Schapiro MB, Grady CL, et al: Cerebral glucose metabolism in childhood-onset obsessive-compulsive disorder. Arch Gen Psychiatry 46:518–523, 1989

Szymanski HV: Prolonged depersonalization after marijuana abuse. Am J Psychiatry 138:231–233, 1981

Thomas CS: Dysmorphophobia: a question of definition. Br J Psychiatry 144:513–516, 1984

Thomas CS: Dysmorphophobia and monosymptomatic hypochondriasis (letter). Am J Psychiatry 142:1121, 1985

Thomas CS: Anorexia nervosa and dysmorphophobia (letter). Br J Psychiatry 150:406, 1987

Thorén P, Åsberg M, Cronholm B, et al: Clomipramine treatment of obsessive-compulsive disorder, I: a controlled clinical trial. Arch Gen Psychiatry 37:1281–1285, 1980a

Thorén P, Åsberg M, Bertilsson L, et al: Clomipramine treatment of obsessive-compulsive disorder, II: biochemical aspects. Arch Gen Psychiatry 37:1289–1294, 1980b

Torch EM: Review of the relationship between obsession and depersonalization. Acta Psychiatr Scand 58:191–198, 1978

Torch EM: Depersonalization syndrome: an overview. Psychiatr Q 53:249–258, 1981

Tucker GJ, Harrow M, Quinlan D: Depersonalization, dysphoria, and thought disturbance. Am J Psychiatry 130:702–706, 1973

Turner SM, Jacob RG, Morrison R: Somatoform and factitious disorders, in Comprehensive Handbook of Psychopathology. Edited by Adams HE, Sutker PB. New York, Plenum, 1984, pp 307–345

Vitiello B, DeLeon J: Dysmorphophobia misdiagnosed as obsessive-compulsive disorder. Psychosomatics 31:220–222, 1990

Walsh RN: Depersonalization: definition and treatment (letter). Am J Psychiatry 132:873, 1975

Winokur G: Delusional disorder (paranoia). Compr Psychiatry 18:511–521, 1977

Zohar J, Mueller EA, Insel TR, et al: Serotonergic responsivity in obsessive-compulsive disorder. Arch Gen Psychiatry 44:946–951, 1987

Zohar J, Insel TR, Zohar-Kadouch RC, et al: Serotonergic responsivity in obsessive-compulsive disorder: effects of chronic clomipramine treatment. Arch Gen Psychiatry 45:167–172, 1988

Chapter 3

Anorexia Nervosa

Walter H. Kaye, M.D.
Theodore Weltzin, M.D.
L. K. George Hsu, M.D.

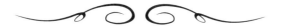

Anorexia nervosa, a disorder of unknown etiology, most commonly occurs in adolescent females. According to DSM-III-R
(American Psychiatric Association 1987), anorexia nervosa is characterized by several essential features (see Table 3–1):

1. A refusal to maintain body weight over a minimal weight normal
   for age and height
2. An intense fear of gaining weight or of becoming fat, even though
   underweight
3. A disturbance in the way in which one's body weight, size, or
   shape is experienced (e.g., the person claims to "feel fat" even
   when emaciated)

Most anorexic individuals have a marked diminution of food
intake in the obsessive pursuit of thinness. Some persons with this
disorder have binge episodes usually followed by purging. In addition, anorexic individuals display a stereotypic rigidity, ritualism,
perfectionism, and meticulousness. It is noted in DSM-III-R that
compulsive behaviors, such as hand washing, may be present and

Table 3–1.   DSM-III-R criteria for anorexia nervosa (307.10)

1. Refusal to maintain body weight over a minimal normal weight for age and height, e.g., weight loss leading to maintenance of body weight 15% below that expected; or failure to make expected weight gain during period of growth, leading to body weight 15% below that expected.
2. Intense fear of gaining weight or becoming fat, even though underweight.
3. Disturbance in the way in which one's body weight, size, or shape is experienced, e.g., the person claims to "feel fat" even when emaciated, believes that one area of the body is "too fat" even when obviously underweight.
4. In females, absence of at least three consecutive menstrual cycles when otherwise expected to occur (primary or secondary amenorrhea). (A woman is considered to have amenorrhea if her periods occur only following hormone, e.g., estrogen, administration.)

Source. Reprinted with permission from American Psychiatric Association: *Diagnostic and Statistical Manual of Mental Disorders,* 3rd Edition, Revised. Washington, DC, American Psychiatric Association, 1987. Copyright 1987, American Psychiatric Association.

may justify the additional diagnosis of obsessive-compulsive disorder (OCD). Depression and/or anxiety are often present (Hudson et al. 1983). However, these symptoms may not be readily apparent, as anorexic persons usually deny or minimize the severity of their illness and are uninterested in, or resistant to, therapy.

A typical presentation of anorexia nervosa is given below:

A 13-year-old girl is dragged by her distraught mother into a therapist's office. The mother, who is frightened and upset, explains that her daughter is preoccupied with thoughts of being too fat and is determined to become thin. Her 5-foot-tall daughter weighed about 100 pounds before the onset of these behaviors. Despite the fact that the daughter now is 75 pounds, she still sees herself as too fat and wants to lose more weight. Having begun dieting about 6 months prior to the initial visit, the daughter is now restricting herself to one or two vegetarian, low-fat meals per day, which she eats very slowly and in isolation. Despite this restrictive food intake, she has become obsessed with food, cookbooks, recipes, and cooking for others. In fact, she likes to read recipes or wander through the supermarket looking at food items. At the same time, the daughter describes being frightened of eating and is scared, at times, that actions involving nonfood items, such as putting on cold cream, will cause weight gain.

The mother describes escalating battles at home between herself and her daughter, not only over eating and weight loss but over almost any decision or normal detail of life. She describes her daughter as becoming increasingly argumentative and rigid. When wanting something, her daughter will pester and fret over this issue until the mother gives in just to get some peace and quiet. In addition, her daughter has become increasingly isolated from her friends and has become overly serious, with little interest in having fun.

While always a good student, the daughter has become even more studious and concerned with her grades. She re-reads assignments and copies homework over until it is perfect. The mother also mentions that her daughter spends several hours a day cleaning the house or her own bedroom and that everything in her daughter's bedroom is neat and in a certain order—for example, all the clothes in her closet are ordered by color. As her mother points out, the daughter feels that she must exercise daily, usually for an hour. In addition, she walks 2 miles to and from school and rarely sits. In fact, she seems like she is in constant motion because of fidgeting or additional exercising such as unnecessary deep knee bends. The mother describes her child as always having been a "model child" who did things right and rarely got into trouble.

When the daughter is interviewed alone, she appears to be relatively unconcerned with why her mother is making her come to see a therapist. The daughter explains, "There is nothing wrong with me; I'm just too fat and I'll feel better if I lose another 5 pounds." When asked to explain her mother's concerns, the daughter states that "she is just jealous of my ability to lose weight" and that "Mom is lying when she says I'm too thin." With another line of questioning, the daughter comments that she wants "to be perfect but that she feels that she is not perfect enough." She also indicates that she expects other people to be perfect and that she is constantly irritated by the fact that other people do not live up to her expectation of perfection.

We have limited understanding of the reasons why anorexic individuals have such symptomatology. Psychodynamic theories have suggested that such symptoms are the result of conflicts concerning the family, difficulties with psychosexual development, or sociocultural influences. More recently, it has been suggested that anorexia nervosa may be related to major affective disorders. These theories, however, do not really explain the meaning of anorectic symptoms such as body image distortion, pathological feeding behavior, perfectionism, or compulsive exercise. It has been suggested for at least the last 50 years that anorexia nervosa has some relationship to obsessive and compulsive behaviors. In this regard, the inherently obsessional nature of anorexia nervosa is obvious, with obsessional calorie counting, body preoccupation, and incessant ruminations about food. In this chapter we present lines of evidence that support the hypothesis that there is some link between anorexia nervosa and obsessionality and/or compulsivity. We first will review the studies that have assessed obsessionality in anorexia nervosa. We then will examine the limited literature suggesting an increased incidence of prior anorexia nervosa in patients who present with OCD.

It should be noted that, compared with other psychiatric disorders, anorexia nervosa is a relatively homogeneous illness in terms of the person's age at onset, gender of vulnerability, and symptom complex. The remarkable degree of consistency in the clinical presentation of anorexic patients could be due to a malfunction of some neurobiological systems, such as brain serotonergic systems. Thus, we will review neurochemical and psychopharmacological data suggesting that a disturbance of serotonin activity could be the link that cuts across the diagnostic boundaries of anorexia nervosa and OCD.

Studies of Comorbidity

Depression

Studies of comorbidity in anorexia nervosa have examined the presence of concomitant psychopathology during the acute phase of the illness and following short- and long-term recovery. Perhaps the most widely reported comorbid feature of anorexia nervosa is depression, with estimates that 21% to 91% of patients have depressive symptomatology during the acute phase of anorexia (Eckert et al. 1982; Hendren 1983; Morgan and Russell 1975; Stonehill and Crisp 1977; Theander 1970). When interpreting these findings, one must consider that common behavioral accompaniments of starvation (Keys 1950; Strober 1988) closely resemble the accessory symptoms of primary depressive disorder and, thus, may inflate depression rating scores in underweight anorexic patients.

The presence of depressive symptomatology has also been examined in anorexic patients after short- and long-term weight recovery (Strober 1988). With duration of follow-up ranging from several months to 4.9 years, an estimated 15% to 58% of patients continued to exhibit some degree of depressive disturbance after weight recovery. These widely varying estimates reflect differential methodological and diagnostic procedures across studies. It is important to note that there has been much controversy as to whether anorexia nervosa and major depression share a common diathesis. Critical examination of clinical phenomenology, family history, antidepressant response, biological correlates, course and outcome, and epidemiology yields *limited* support for this hypothesis (Strober 1988).

The Relationship Between Anorexia Nervosa and Obsessive-Compulsive Disorder

The focus on the possible relationship between depression and anorexia nervosa has obscured investigations of other associated psychopathology. In fact, patients with anorexia nervosa have a high prevalence of obsessive-compulsive symptoms or of OCD (Cantwell et al. 1977; Hsu et al. 1979; Rothenberg 1988; Rowland 1970; Strober 1980) as well other anxiety disorders (Toner et al. 1986). For example, Hudson and co-workers (1983) reported that 81% of restricter anorexic patients and 92% of bulimic anorexic patients had a history of an affective disorder during their lifetime. However, these authors also found that the restricter and bulimic subgroups had a 75% and 56% incidence of anxiety disorders, respectively, with a 69% and 44% incidence of OCD.

Descriptive studies.   Early descriptive investigations of personality characteristics beginning more than 50 years ago performed on individuals with anorexia nervosa highlighted the finding that these individuals tend to be rigid, perfectionistic, and obsessional (Palmer and Jones 1939). Dubois (1949) suggested that anorexia nervosa be renamed "compulsion neurosis with cachexia." Then, in a series of studies involving patients with anorexia nervosa, a high incidence of obsessional traits was reported. Kay and Leigh (1954) reported that 50% of 38 anorexic patients had premorbid obsessional traits. King (1963) found that all of their 12 anorexic patients had obsessional features, and Dally (1969) found that 81% of 140 anorexic patients had obsessional personalities. On the other hand, Morgan and Russell (1975) found that only 27% of anorexic patients in their sample had obsessional premorbid personalities. Finally, Norris (1979) found that 60% of 54 anorexic patients had premorbid obsessionality.

Rothenberg (1988) compiled data from 11 major investigations of comorbidity in anorexia nervosa. He concluded that obsessive-compulsive symptoms were the second most frequently reported symptoms after those of depression. Between 11% and 83% of patients displayed obsessive-compulsive features during acute anorexia nervosa or after weight restoration. Rothenberg hypothesizes that the depression seen in anorexia nervosa may be secondary to a more intrinsic relationship with obsessive-compulsive symptoms rather than a primary association between anorexia nervosa and affective disorders.

In another review, Holden (1990) found that premorbid obsessional personality traits are overrepresented in those patients with anorexia nervosa. However, he concludes that the illness process, especially starvation, serves to exaggerate these traits so that further conclusions are speculative.

Psychological assessments. Controlled studies have found anorexic patients to be significantly more neurotic, less extraverted, and more anxious than control subjects (Smart et al. 1976). Solyom and colleagues (1982) found that individuals with anorexia nervosa display high trait scores on inventories assessing obsessive-compulsive features and that the scores of the anorexic patients were comparable to those of matched patients with OCD. The authors concluded that approximately one-half of their anorexic patients would qualify for a diagnosis of OCD, even after excluding food- and body-related obsessions.

We evaluated a sample of anorexic patients for the presence of OCD-like symptoms (after excluding core anorexic traits) using the Yale-Brown Obsessive Compulsive Scale (Y-BOCS) (Goodman et al. 1989b, 1989c) (see Table 3–2), a recently developed semistructured interview designed to rate the severity and type of symptoms in patients with OCD. We found that 19 unmedicated anorexic patients had a mean score of 22 ± 5 on the Y-BOCS, which was similar in magnitude to the mean score reported by Goodman and colleagues (1989c) for 81 OCD patients (25 ± 6) and Jenike and colleagues (1989) for 61 OCD patients (22 ± 6). Moreover, anorexic and control patients had no crossover in the range of their Y-BOCS scores. Every anorexic patient had OCD-like symptoms, even when the core symptoms (body-image distortion, pathological feeding, and exercise) typical of

Table 3–2. Percentage of anorexia nervosa patients ($n = 19$) endorsing specific obsessional and compulsive behaviors on the Yale-Brown Obsessive Compulsive Scale symptom checklist

Category[a]	Type[b]	Percentage
OBS	Fear of not saying things right	73
OBS	Fear of doing something embarrassing	68
OBS	Preoccupation with symmetry, exactness	55
OBS	Need to know, remember	55
COMP	Clean household, inanimate objects	55
OBS	Fear something terrible will happen	55
OBS	Responsible that things will go wrong	50
COMP	Ordering/arranging compulsions	45
OBS	Fear saying certain words or phrases	45
COMP	Excessive or ritualized bathing, grooming	45
OBS	Preoccupation with hoarding/collecting	41
OBS	Concern with dirt, germs	41
OBS	Afraid of blurting obscenities, insults	36
OBS/COMP	Somatic preoccupation and rituals	23
COMP	Excessive, ritualized hand washing	23
OBS	Fear of harming self	23
OBS	Religious obsessions	18
COMP	Counting compulsions	18
OBS	Concern about household items	18
OBS	Worries that others will get ill	18

[a]OBS = obsessive; COMP = compulsive.
[b]See Goodman et al. 1989b, 1989c.

anorexia nervosa were *excluded*. Anorexic patients had 10 ± 5 (range: 3 to 21) individual obsessive and compulsive symptoms on the Y-BOCS checklist. The 20 most frequently endorsed individual symptoms on the checklist are shown in Table 3–2. Fourteen of these items were obsessions. In contrast, 38 of the obsessive or compulsive items on the checklist were infrequently endorsed: 5 of the obsessive or compulsive items on the checklist were endorsed by only three anorexic patients (14%), 6 items by two anorexic patients (9%), 13 items by only one anorexic patient (5%), and 14 items by no anorexic patients. These 38 infrequently endorsed obsessions and compulsions on the Y-BOCS checklist were primarily composed of checking compulsions, repeating rituals, and sexual obsessions. Importantly, there was no difference in Y-BOCS scores between underweight and weight-restored anorexic patients. We found, as did Rothenberg (1986), that anorexic patients had particular concerns with ordering and cleanliness, or an obsession with perfectionism or with things going wrong.

State versus trait. Invariably, investigations of personality traits performed during the acute phase of anorexia nervosa are strongly influenced by the subject's malnutrition and the presence of pathophysiological disturbances. Some studies have tried to determine the effects of weight loss and nutrition on personality functioning by reassessing anorexic patients after recent attainment of weight recovery or after long-term weight recovery. Stonehill and Crisp (1977) found that underweight anorexic patients scored significantly higher than control patients on anxiety, obsessional, somatic, and depression scales, with no difference in phobic and hysterical scores. After being re-fed a short while before, weight-restoration anorexic patients showed significantly lower somatic scores and trends toward lower anxiety and obsessional scores, while extraversion was significantly elevated and neuroticism was significantly decreased. Twenty-nine patients were assessed 4 to 7 years later and were found to have significantly higher phobia and hysteria scores than they did before treatment. The authors concluded that as long as the phobic focus of the anorexic patient is on her weight, her social phobia is not manifest; however, as she abandons the "psychological avoidance of adolescence," the anorexic patient is faced with increased social demands, and her social anxiety and phobias emerge.

Similar results were found by Strober (1980), who studied 22 nonchronic adolescents at presentation and after short-term (i.e., recently re-fed) weight recovery. At short-term follow-up there was increased extraversion; a decrease in symptom, but not trait, obsessionality; and decreased drive for social approval. Most interesting was the persistence of obsessional traits after weight restoration. Strober characterized recovered anorexic patients as obsessional, with inflexible thinking, social introversion, overly compliant behavior, and limited social spontaneity. The author suggested that those underlying traits may play a facilitating role in the development of obsessive and compulsive symptoms during the acute illness.

Casper (1990) more recently reported that women who were recovered from restricting anorexia nervosa for 8 to 10 years continued to have inhibited behavior. That is, such women rated higher on risk avoidance, displayed greater restraint in emotional expression and initiative, and showed greater conformance to authority than did age-matched control subjects. They also had a greater degree of self-control and impulse control than their sisters.

Comparison of restricter and bulimic anorexic patients. Considerable literature (Beaumont et al. 1976; Casper et al. 1980; Garfinkel et al. 1980; Garner et al. 1985; Halmi and Falk 1982; Herzog and Copeland 1985; Strober et al. 1982) suggests that patients with anorexia nervosa can be subdivided by certain variables, including type of pathological eating behavior and psychopathological characteristics. The terminology used to differentiate these subgroups has been in flux. Specifically, *restricter,* or fasting, anorexic patients (who tend to fit the DSM-III-R criteria for anorexia nervosa alone) lose weight by pure dieting. *Bulimic* anorexic patients (who qualify for a DSM-III-R diagnosis of both anorexia nervosa and bulimia nervosa) also lose weight but have a periodic disinhibition of restraint and engage in bingeing and purging. Compared with restricter patients, the bulimic subgroup has been characterized as displaying significantly more evidence of premorbid behavioral instability, a higher incidence of premorbid and familial obesity, a greater susceptibility to depression, and a higher incidence of behaviors suggestive of impulse disorder.

Strober (1980) noted that bulimic anorexic patients were more socially adept and exhibited greater impairment of self-control mechanisms than did restricter anorexic patients. However, he noted certain commonalities between these two subgroups, including obsessional characteristics, heightened industriousness and responsibility, interpersonal insecurity, minimization of affect, and excessive conformance and regimentation of behavior.

Genetic and epidemiologic studies. There have been few family epidemiologic studies of the coaggregation of eating disorders and other psychiatric illnesses. The few that have been done have mainly studied the coexistence of affective disorders. Strober and colleagues (1990), in a large and well-controlled family epidemiologic study of anorexia nervosa, found an excess of affective disorders (mainly unipolar) among relatives of only the anorexic probands who were themselves depressed. Biederman's group (1985) had similar findings. In contrast, Gershon and colleagues (1984) found equally high rates of affective disorder among relatives of depressed and nondepressed anorexic probands.

A few studies have used more rigorous family study methods to compare the lifetime rate of eating disorders among relatives of anorexic patients and relatives of normal control subjects. All of these studies have shown an increased occurrence of eating disorders in the relatives of probands with eating disorders. Gershon and colleagues (1984) found a familial aggregation of eating disorders, with nearly a sixfold increase in risk of this disorder among relatives of anorexic probands. Strober and colleagues (1990) found that anorexia nervosa clustered in families, suggesting intergenerational transmission.

Two studies of anorexia nervosa involving twins have found that proband concordance was significantly higher for monozygotic pairs than it was for dizygotic pairs (0.66–0.71 vs. 0.10–0.25, respectively) (Holland et al. 1984, 1988). Estimates of heritability based on these data ranged from 0.54 to 0.98, whereas nongenetic familial and environmental effects accounted for only 0.02 to 0.38 of the variance in liability.

To our knowledge, no family studies assessing the prevalence of OCD or anxiety disorders in the relatives of anorexic probands have been done. Several investigators (Kasvikis et al. 1986; T. R. Insel, personal communication, September 1985) have noted that adult women with OCD have an increased incidence of prior anorexia nervosa. However, no studies, to our knowledge, have systematically assessed the prevalence of anorexia nervosa in the relatives of probands with anxiety disorders or OCD.

Overview. It is not clear whether anorexia nervosa is a variant of OCD or is a distinct disorder that shares some common symptoms. Nevertheless, numerous data suggest that individuals with anorexia nervosa show considerable obsessive symptomatology, above and beyond that directly related to the eating disturbance.

Central Nervous System Serotonin Activity

Elevated CSF 5-HIAA in Long-Term Weight-Restored Anorexic Patients

Considerable data in animals and humans implicate brain serotonergic systems in the modulation of appetite, mood, personality variables, and neuroendocrine function. Thus, a brain serotonergic dysfunction could contribute to many aspects of the anorexia nervosa symptom complex.

To avoid the confounding influences of malnutrition or weight loss, we studied patients with anorexia nervosa at normal weight and stable dietary intake (Kaye et al. 1991a). Compared with control subjects, long-term weight-restored anorexic patients had elevated concentrations of cerebrospinal fluid (CSF) 5-hydroxyindoleacetic acid (5-HIAA), the major serotonin metabolite, whereas levels of CSF homovanillic acid (HVA), the major dopamine metabolite, were normal. Elevated levels of CSF 5-HIAA may indicate increased serotonin activity. These data are of interest because most anorexic patients have ingrained traits of psychopathology that are consistent with a possible intrinsic disturbance of serotonin activity.

Considerable evidence shows that brain serotonergic pathways are inhibitory of appetite. In terms of appetitive behaviors, treatments that increase intrasynaptic serotonin or directly activate serotonin receptors tend to reduce food consumption (Blundell 1984; Leibowitz and Shor-Posner 1986; Wurtman and Wurtman 1979). Conversely, interventions that diminish serotonergic neurotransmissions or serotonin receptor activation reportedly increase food consumption and promote weight gain. Theoretically, food restriction and weight loss could be caused by increased serotonin activity. Kaye et al.'s (1991a) study raises the provocative question of whether anorexic subjects have an alteration in serotonin activity that contributes to a trait toward pathological feeding behavior and weight loss.

As noted above, anorexia nervosa patients are rigid, ritualistic, perfectionistic, and meticulous. Considerable studies have found that low levels of CSF 5-HIAA are associated with impulsive, suicidal, and aggressive behavior (Åsberg et al. 1976; Brown et al. 1979; Linnoila et al. 1983; van Praag 1983). Thus, higher levels of CSF 5-HIAA in long-term weight-restored anorexic patients are of interest because these patients tend to be the opposite of impulsive and aggressive patients.

Several lines of evidence support the possibility of an abnormality of serotonin activity in OCD. The most compelling evidence is that serotonin-specific medications are effective in the treatment of OCD (Ananth et al. 1981; Goodman et al. 1989a; Perse et al. 1987; Thorén et al. 1980b; Volavka et al. 1985). Zohar and colleagues (1988) and Hollander's group (1991) found that clomipramine and fluoxetine, respectively, induced adaptive down-regulation of serotonergic responsiveness in patients with OCD. These studies support the possibility that increased serotonergic responsiveness is associated with the psychopathological characteristics of OCD. In terms of CSF 5-HIAA, higher concentrations have been found in one group of OCD patients (Insel et al. 1985) but not another (Thorén et al. 1980a). In the latter study, OCD patients appeared to have a bimodal distribution of CSF 5-HIAA concentrations, because OCD patients responding to clomipramine had higher pretreatment CSF 5-HIAA levels.

Increased serotonin activity may contribute to overly inhibited behavior in animals and to obsessive and anxious behavior in humans. Soubrie (1986) suggested that serotonergic neurons are involved in enabling the organism to arrange or tolerate delay before acting. Cloninger (1987) suggested that serotonergic neuronal systems are an important component of behavioral inhibition, specifically harm avoidance. Preclinical (Charney et al. 1987) and clinical (Cloninger 1987; Kahn et al. 1988) studies suggest that increased activity of serotonergic neuronal systems appears to be involved in anxiety disorders (Howard and Pollard 1977), and drugs with pronounced effects on serotonergic systems have been reported to be useful for the treatment of generalized anxiety disorder (Leysen et al. 1985; Taylor et al. 1985).

Taken together, reduced serotonin transmission may produce a lower inhibition of behavioral response, whereas increased serotonin transmission may overly inhibit behavioral response and/or increase anxiety. We hypothesize that increased serotonin activity is associated with certain characteristics, such as rigidity, anxiety, inhibition, or obsessional behaviors, that cut across the boundaries of diagnostic categories.

Differences in CSF 5-HIAA Accumulation Between Restricter and Bulimic Anorexic Patients

We have reported (Kaye et al. 1984) that after probenecid infusion, weight-recovered nonbulimic anorexic patients had higher levels of CSF 5-HIAA than did bulimic anorexic patients. However, we have found no difference between anorexic subtypes in a morning baseline study (i.e., a nonprobenecid study). We cannot discount the possibility that alterations in postprobenecid CSF 5-HIAA levels might be due to differences in membrane transport characteristics between bulimic and nonbulimic anorexic patients, to the central effects of probenecid itself (Cowdry et al. 1983), or to diurnal variations in CSF 5-HIAA levels. Alternatively, an 8-hour probenecid-induced accumulation of CSF 5-HIAA might provide a greater degree of precision in terms of measurement of serotonin turnover in the central nervous system than does a baseline lumbar puncture. Taken together, these data suggest that increased serotonin activity could contribute to certain attributes found in both restricter and bulimic anorexic patients, including obsessional and overly inhibited characteristics, as well as the pursuit of thinness. Alternatively, it is possible that restricter and bulimic anorexic patients exist along a continuum, with restricters having relatively greater serotonin activity than do bulimic anorexic patients, as evidenced by the fact that the latter have cyclical and episodic behavioral patterns manifested by swings from impulsivity to compulsivity.

The Effects of Serotonin-Specific Medication in Anorexia Nervosa

The possibility of some relationship between anorexia nervosa and OCD raised the question of how anorexic patients would respond to a serotonin-specific medication. In fact, some evidence shows that medications with serotonergic properties have some efficacy in the treatment of anorexia nervosa. Crisp and colleagues (1987) administered clomipramine, a serotonin reuptake blocker, to anorexic patients engaged in a program of re-feeding and weight gain and found it to be associated with increased appetite, hunger, and caloric consumption during the early stages of treatment. Halmi and colleagues (1986) found that restricter anorexic patients had a better response than bulimic anorexic patients to cyproheptadine, a serotonin antagonist. Our group (Kaye et al. 1991b) has treated 31 anorexic patients with an open trial of fluoxetine, a serotonin reuptake blocker that is effective in the treatment of OCD. Response was good in 11 and partial in another 16 anorexic patients as measured by the fact that all of these patients were able to maintain a weight of greater than 85% ABW in 10 ± 7 months as outpatients and showed improvements in eating behavior, mood, and obsessional symptoms. In these preliminary data, we have also found that restricters responded significantly better to a medication with serotonergic properties than did bulimic/purging anorexic patients.

Anorexia, OCD, and Obsessive-Compulsive Personality Traits

The relationship between symptoms in anorexia nervosa and symptoms in OCD remains undefined. It should be noted that the

DSM-III-R superficially addresses the issue of the overlap of anorexia nervosa and OCD. The DSM-III-R notes that compulsive behaviors may be present in anorexia nervosa and may justify an additional diagnosis of OCD. To diagnose someone with OCD, according to the DSM-III-R, if an eating disorder occurs in the patient, the content of the obsession should not be related to symptoms specific to an eating disorder such as food.

Since the DSM-III-R was published, accumulating data raise new questions about the relationship of anorexia nervosa and OCD. First, there is the question of whether core anorexic symptoms, per se, are obsessive and compulsive behaviors as defined by DSM-III-R. That is, are body-image distortion and pursuit of thinness forms of obsessional thoughts, and are pathological feeding and exercise forms of compulsive behaviors? Second, do anorexic patients have typical OCD symptoms that are distinct from core anorexic symptoms, such as preoccupation with dirt or germs or repeated hand washing. Third, do anorexic patients have personality traits that are similar to DSM-III-R obsessive-compulsive personality disorder? Fourth, are these symptoms secondary to weight loss or malnutrition, or are they an intrinsic disturbance central to the development of this illness?

Are Anorexic Symptoms Forms of Obsessions and Compulsions as Defined by DSM-III-R?

In our opinion, anorexic core symptoms resemble obsessions and compulsions in many ways. Anorexic patients have recurrent, persistent, and intrusive thoughts about their body image and desire for thinness. Furthermore, anorexia nervosa patients recognize that the obsessions are the product of their own mind. However, obsessions are defined in DSM-III-R as senseless thoughts or impulses that the person attempts to ignore or suppress or to neutralize with some other thought or action. At the onset of their illness, most anorexic patients do not regard core symptoms as senseless and often do not attempt to ignore or suppress these thoughts. Only after treatment do some anorexic patients begin to regard thoughts about their body image as senseless.

As regards compulsions, anorexic patients persistently exercise and have odd, ritualized eating behaviors. These behaviors resemble compulsions because they are repetitive, purposeful, and intentional and are performed in response to an obsession or in accordance with certain rules or in a stereotyped fashion. However, anorexic patients may be different from patients with OCD in that the intent of anorexic compulsions may not be to neutralize or prevent discomfort. In addition, the majority of anorexic patients do not recognize that such behaviors are excessive or unreasonable. However, it must be noted that in the DSM-III-R it is stated that young children or those with overvalued ideas may not recognize that such behaviors are excessive or unreasonable. The issue of whether or not core anorexic symptoms are a variant of OCD remains controversial. An alternative hypothesis is that anorexic patients and patients with OCD may share certain common neurobiological abnormalities that cut across traditional diagnostic boundaries and contribute to similar psychopathological processes that have certain differences in terms of content.

Do Anorexic Patients Have Typical OCD Behaviors That Are Independent of Core Anorexic Symptoms?

Limited data show that anorexic patients do have typical OCD behaviors that are independent of core anorexic symptoms (Rothenberg 1986; Solyom et al. 1982; Strober 1988). There are several reasons why frequent and severe OCD-like symptoms in anorexic patients have not been more readily recognized. First, certain behaviors that might attract attention, such as checking compulsions, are usually not present in anorexic patients. Second, many of the frequent obsessions, such as fear of embarrassment or of doing something wrong, may have been discounted as typical of anorexia nervosa but not thought of as OCD symptoms. Third, such symptoms may be overshadowed by the intensity of the core anorexia nervosa symptoms such as devotion to thinness. Fourth, and most importantly, we have been struck, as were Solyom et al. (1982) and others, by the fact that anorexic patients minimize or deny OCD-like symptoms. For example, in our hospital, one patient who washed her hands more than 40 times per day (to the extent that her hands were red and cracked) would offer a plausible explanation for each hand-washing episode and did not regard this behavior as abnormal. Such symptoms, therefore, appear to be ego-syntonic in anorexic patients, in contrast to the ego-dystonic symptoms more commonly, but not always, found in OCD patients. In this regard, anorexic core symptoms, such as feeling fat when underweight, are also ego-syntonic, and anorexic patients will vigorously deny that such symptoms are abnormal.

Do Anorexic Patients Have Obsessive-Compulsive Personality Disorder?

Patients with anorexia nervosa often are perfectionistic, are preoccupied with details, have an unreasonable insistence that others submit to exactly their way of doing things, have excessive devotion to work and productivity (often school), are overconscientious, and have restricted expression of affection. To our knowledge no studies have formally tested the hypothesis that such symptoms meet criteria for DSM-III-R obsessive-compulsive personality disorder using a structured questionnaire (such as the Structured Clinical Interview for DSM-III-R) in a blind manner.

Obsessive-Compulsive Behaviors in Anorexia Nervosa Malnourished State or Trait Related?

While the relationship of obsessive and compulsive behaviors to a malnourished state has not been extensively studied, several studies (Casper 1990; Strober 1980) suggest that such traits endure in anorexic patients after recovery from weight loss. It can be argued that persistent inhibited and rigid personality factors are secondary to chronic malnutrition or overlearned behaviors. However, the persistence of these traits after recovery raises a question as to whether such behaviors contribute to the pathogenesis of this illness.

Summary

There is a growing body of literature that suggests that there are both clinical and biological similarities between anorexia nervosa and

OCD. At this point we are only beginning to understand how the obsessive-compulsive symptoms in anorexia nervosa compare with those seen in OCD. However, a better understanding of this relationship is important for two reasons. First, there is a need to formulate testable hypotheses for understanding the behavioral expression of biological (serotonergic) systems that are dysregulated across psychopathological states. Second, this new understanding may point to new ways of treating this intractable illness. That is, a considerable literature suggests that both serotonin-specific medications and behavioral therapies are useful for treating patients with OCD. Thus, it is possible that such therapies could be adapted for the treatment of patients with anorexia nervosa.

References

American Psychiatric Association: Diagnostic and Statistical Manual of Mental Disorders, 3rd Edition, Revised. Washington, DC, American Psychiatric Association, 1987

Ananth J, Pecknold JC, Van der Steen N, et al: Double-blind comparative study of clomipramine and amitriptyline in obsessive neurosis. Prog Neuropsychopharmacol Biol Psychiatry 5:257–262, 1981

Åsberg M, Träskman L, Thorén P: 5-HIAA in the cerebrospinal fluid: a biochemical suicide predictor? Arch Gen Psychiatry 33:1193–1197, 1976

Beaumont PJV, George GCW, Smart DE: 'Dieters' and 'vomiters' in anorexia nervosa. Psychol Med 6:617–622, 1976

Biederman J, Rivinus T, Kemper K, et al: Depressive disorders in relatives of anorexia nervosa patients with and without a current episode of nonbipolar major depression. Am J Psychiatry 142:1495–1497, 1985

Blundell JE: Serotonin and appetite. Neuropharmacology 23:1537–1551, 1984

Brown GL, Goodwin FK, Ballenger JC, et al: Aggression in humans correlates with cerebrospinal fluid amine metabolites. Psychiatry Res 1:131–139, 1979

Cantwell DP, Sturzenberger, Burroughs J, et al: Anorexia nervosa: an affective disorder? Arch Gen Psychiatry 34:1087–1093, 1977

Casper RC: Personality features of women with good outcome from restricting anorexia nervosa. Psychosom Med 52:156–170, 1990

Casper RC, Eckert ED, Halmi KA, et al: Bulimia: its incidence and clinical importance in patients with anorexia nervosa. Arch Gen Psychiatry 37:1030–1035, 1980

Charney DS, Woods SW, Goodman WK, et al: Serotonin function in anxiety. Psychopharmacology (Berlin) 92:14–24, 1987

Cloninger CR: Neurogenic adaptive mechanism in alcoholism. Science 235:410–416, 1987

Cowdry RW, Ebert MH, van Kammen DP, et al: Cerebrospinal fluid probenecid studies: a reinterpretation. Biol Psychiatry 18:1287–1299, 1983

Crisp AH, Lacey JH, Crutchfield M: Clomipramine and 'drive' in people with anorexia nervosa: an inpatient study. Br J Psychiatry 150:355–358, 1987

Dally P: Anorexia Nervosa. Philadelphia, PA, Grune & Stratton, 1969

DuBois FS: Compulsion neurosis with cachexia (anorexia nervosa). Am J Psychiatry 106:107–115, 1949

Eckert ED, Goldberg SC, Halmi KA, et al: Depression in anorexia nervosa. Psychol Med 12:115–122, 1982

Garfinkel PE, Moldofsky H, Garner DM: The heterogeneity of anorexia nervosa: bulimia as a distinct subgroup. Arch Gen Psychiatry 37:1036–1040, 1980

Garner DM, Garfinkel PE, O'Shaughnessy M: The validity of the distinction between bulimia with and without anorexia nervosa. Am J Psychiatry 142:581–587, 1985

Gershon ES, Schreiber JL, Hamovit JR, et al: Clinical findings in patients with anorexia nervosa and affective illness in their relatives. Am J Psychiatry 141:1419–1422, 1984

Goodman WK, Price LH, Rasmussen SA, et al: Efficacy of fluvoxamine in obsessive-compulsive disorder: a double-blind comparison with placebo. Arch Gen Psychiatry 46:36–44, 1989a

Goodman WK, Price LH, Rasmussen SA, et al: The Yale-Brown Obsessive Compulsive Scale, I: development, use, and reliability. Arch Gen Psychiatry 46:1006–1011, 1989b

Goodman WK, Price LH, Rasmussen SA, et al: The Yale-Brown Obsessive Compulsive Scale, II: validity. Arch Gen Psychiatry 46:1012–1016, 1989c

Halmi KA, Falk JR: Anorexia nervosa: a study of outcome discriminators in exclusive dieters and bulimics. Journal of the American Academy of Child Psychiatry 21:369–375, 1982

Halmi KA, Eckert ED, LaDu TJ, et al: Anorexia nervosa: treatment efficacy of cyproheptadine and amitriptyline. Arch Gen Psychiatry 43:177–181, 1986

Hendren RL: Depression in anorexia nervosa. Journal of the American Academy of Child Psychiatry 22:59–62, 1983

Herzog DB, Copeland PM: Eating disorders. N Engl J Med 313:295–303, 1985

Holden NL: Is anorexia nervosa an obsessive-compulsive disorder? Br J Psychiatry 157:1–5, 1990

Holland AJ, Hall A, Murray R, et al: Anorexia nervosa: a study of 34 twin pairs and one set of triplets. Br J Psychiatry 145:414–419, 1984

Holland AJ, Sicotte N, Treasure J: Anorexia nervosa: evidence for a genetic basis. J Psychosomat Res 32:561–571, 1988

Hollander E, DeCaria C, Gully R, et al: Effects of chronic fluoxetine treatment on behavioral and neuroendocrine responses to meta-chloro-phenylpiperazine in obsessive-compulsive disorder. Psychiatry Res 36:1–17, 1991

Howard JL, Pollard GT: Animal models, in Psychiatry and Neurology. Edited by Kanin I, Usdin E. New York, Pergamon, 1977, pp 269–277

Hsu LKG, Crisp AH, Harding B: Outcome of anorexia nervosa. Lancet 1:61–65, 1979

Hudson JI, Pope HG Jr, Jonas JM, et al: Phenomenologic relationship of eating disorders to major affective disorder. Psychiatry Res 9:345–354, 1983

Insel TR, Mueller EA, Alterman I, et al: Obsessive-compulsive disorder and serotonin: is there a connection? Biol Psychiatry 20:1174–1188, 1985

Jenike MA, Buttolph L, Baer L, et al: Open trial of fluoxetine in obsessive-compulsive disorder. Am J Psychiatry 146:909–911, 1989

Kahn RS, van Praag HM, Wetzler S, et al: Serotonin and anxiety revisited. Biol Psychiatry 23:189–208, 1988

Kasvikis YG, Tsakiris F, Marks IM, et al: Past history of anorexia nervosa in women with obsessive-compulsive disorder. International Journal of Eating Disorders 5:1069–1075, 1986

Kay DW, Leigh D: The natural history, treatment, and prognosis of anorexia nervosa, based on a study of 38 patients. Journal of Mental Science 100:411–431, 1954

Kaye WH, Ebert MH, Gwirtsman HE, et al: Differences in brain serotonergic metabolism between nonbulimic and bulimic patients with anorexia nervosa. Am J Psychiatry 141:1598–1601, 1984

Kaye WH, Gwirtsman HE, George DT, et al: Altered serotonin activity in anorexia nervosa after long-term weight restoration: does elevated cerebrospinal fluid 5-hydroxyindoleacetic acid level correlate with rigid and obsessive behavior? Arch Gen Psychiatry 48:556–562, 1991a

Kaye WH, Weltzin TE, Hsu LKG, et al: An open trial of fluoxetine in patients with anorexia nervosa. J Clin Psychiatry 52:464–471, 1991b

Keys A: The Biology of Human Starvation. Minneapolis, MN, University of Minnesota Press, 1950

King A: Primary and secondary anorexia nervosa syndromes. Br J Psychiatry 109:470–479, 1963

Leibowitz SF, Shor-Posner G: Brain serotonin and eating behavior. Appetite 7:1–14, 1986

Leysen JE, Gommeren W, Van Gompel P: Receptor-binding properties in vitro and in vivo of ritanserin, a very potent and long-acting serotonin-S$_2$ antagonist. Mol Pharmacol 27:600–611, 1985

Linnoila M, Virkkunen M, Scheinin M, et al: Low cerebrospinal fluid 5-HIAA concentration differentiates impulsive from non-impulsive violent behavior. Life Sci 33:2609–2614, 1983

Morgan HG, Russell GFM: Value of family background and clinical features as predictors of long-term outcome in anorexia nervosa: four-year follow-up study of 41 patients. Psychol Med 5:355–371, 1975

Norris DL: Clinical diagnostic criteria for primary anorexia nervosa. S Afr Med J 56:987–993, 1979

Palmer HD, Jones MS: Anorexia nervosa as a manifestation of compulsive neurosis: a study of psychogenic factors. Archives of Neurology and Psychiatry 41:856–860, 1939

Perse TL, Greist JH, Jefferson JW, et al: Fluvoxamine treatment of obsessive-compulsive disorder. Am J Psychiatry 144:1543–1548, 1987

Rothenberg A: Eating disorder as a modern obsessive-compulsive syndrome. Psychiatry 49:45–53, 1986

Rothenberg A: Differential diagnosis of anorexia nervosa and depressive illness: a review of 11 studies. Compr Psychiatry 29:427–432, 1988

Rowland C Jr: Anorexia nervosa: a survey of the literature and review of 30 cases. International Psychiatry Clinics 7:37–137, 1970

Smart DE, Beumont PJV, George GCW: Some personality characteristics of patients with anorexia nervosa. Br J Psychiatry 128:57–60, 1976

Solyom L, Freeman RJ, Miles JE: A comparative psychometric study of anorexia nervosa and obsessive neurosis. Can J Psychiatry 27:282–286, 1982

Soubrie P: Reconciling the role of central serotonin neurosis in human and animal behavior. Behavioral and Brain Sciences 9:319–363, 1986

Stonehill E, Crisp AH: Psychotic characteristics of patients with anorexia nervosa before and after treatment and at follow-up 4–7 years later. J Psychosom Res 21:187–193, 1977

Strober M: Personality and symptomatological features in young, nonchronic anorexia nervosa patients. J Psychosom Res 24:353–359, 1980

Strober M: Depression in the eating disorders: a review and analysis of descriptive, family, and biological findings, in Diagnostic Issues in Anorexia Nervosa and Bulimia Nervosa. Edited by Garner DM, Garfinkel PE. New York, Brunner/Mazel, 1988, pp 80–111

Strober M, Salkin B, Burroughs J, et al: Validity of the bulimia-restricter distinction in anorexia nervosa: parental personality characteristics and family psychiatric morbidity. J Nerv Ment Dis 170:345–351, 1982

Strober M, Lampert C, Morrell W, et al: A controlled family study of anorexia nervosa: evidence of familial aggregation and lack of shared transmission with affective disorders. International Journal of Eating Disorders 9:239–253, 1990

Taylor DP, Eison MDS, Riblet LA: Pharmacological and clinical effects of buspirone. Pharmacol Biochem Behav 23:687–694, 1985

Theander S: Anorexia nervosa: a psychiatric investigation of 94 female patients. Acta Psychiatr Scand Suppl 214:1–194, 1970

Thorén P, Åsberg M, Bertilsson L, et al: Clomipramine treatment of obsessive-compulsive disorder, II: biochemical aspects. Arch Gen Psychiatry 37:1289–1294, 1980a

Thorén P, Åsberg M, Cronholm B, et al: Clomipramine treatment of obsessive-compulsive disorder, I: a controlled clinical trial. Arch Gen Psychiatry 37:1281–1285, 1980b

Toner BB, Garfinkel PE, Garner DM: Long-term follow-up of anorexia nervosa. Psychol Med 48:520–529, 1986

van Praag HM: CSF 5-HIAA and suicide in non-depressed schizophrenics. Lancet 2:977–978, 1983

Volavka J, Neziroglu F, Yaryura-Tobias JA: Clomipramine and imipramine in obsessive-compulsive disorder. Psychiatry Res 14:85–93, 1985

Wurtman JJ, Wurtman RJ: Drugs that enhance central serotoninergic transmission diminish elective carbohydrate consumption by rats. Life Sci 24:895–903, 1979

Zohar J, Insel TR, Zohar-Kadouch RC, et al: Serotonergic responsivity in obsessive-compulsive disorder: effects of chronic clomipramine treatment. Arch Gen Psychiatry 45:167–172, 1988

Chapter 4

Hypochondriasis

Brian A. Fallon, M.D., M.P.H.
Steven A. Rasmussen, M.D.
Michael R. Liebowitz, M.D.

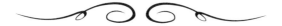

Hypochondriasis is a disorder characterized by obsessions about being ill and compulsions to check with others for either diagnosis and treatment or reassurance that one is not ill. Hypochondriacal individuals, according to the DSM-III-R criteria (American Psychiatric Association 1987), fail to be reassured even if all diagnostic tests and examinations find no evidence of an organic problem. In their obsessions, their compulsions to check, and their failure to be reassured, hypochondriacal individuals are very similar to those persons with obsessive-compulsive disorder (OCD). Is hypochondriasis a variant of OCD? Consider the following cases.

Case 1

Mr. A. is a 33-year-old schoolteacher with a 10-year history of intrusive thoughts about illness. The words "cancer" or "heart attack" enter his mind throughout most of the day, leading to intense anxiety about his health. He tries to neutralize these thoughts by a mental gimmick in which he replaces the word "cancer" with "can't sir" and the words "heart attack" with "heart of gold." At times, he fears other persons are ill when they are not, or that he will infect others with his illness. When unable to neutralize these thoughts or when bodily sensations lead to more intense preoccupation, Mr. A. checks with his doctor for reassurance. Associated symptoms include perfectionism, procrastination, obsessive doubt, and hoarding.

Case 2

Ms. B. is a 28-year-old law student with a 3-year history of fearing that she might have AIDS. Any bodily symptom serves to trigger the fear. A sore throat leads her to wonder: "Is this strep throat or is it AIDS?" She volunteers that her life-style has never placed her at risk for contracting AIDS, yet the fears persist. When reading health law, she feels terrified. She avoids going to the dentist for fear of contamination with AIDS. Although she checks with her boyfriend frequently, Ms. B. rarely checks with doctors, partly because she realizes her fears are irrational and partly because she worries that her worst fears will be confirmed as real. Concurrent diagnoses include body dysmorphic disorder (e.g., "My complexion is unusual—does this mean I have AIDS?") and secondary dysthymia.

Case 3

Ms. C. is a 57-year-old homemaker with a 5-year history of severe hypochondriasis who currently visits her internist once a week because she believes she is suffering from a serious illness. Symptoms began shortly after developing a flu-like illness. Fatigue and myalgia led one doctor to diagnose a systemic yeast infection, and so she has maintained a yeast-free diet; an immunologist, however, subsequently failed to find any signs of a systemic yeast infection. Later, she developed headaches, chest pains, burning sensations in her arms and legs, and extreme vaginal discomfort, which she attempted to treat by cutting a hole in the crotch of her panty hose. Ms. C. has consulted multiple specialists, has received repeated negative diagnostic tests, has been hospitalized twice, and has spent over $100,000 on medical visits and tests. Twenty-three different antidepressants and anxiolytics have each been unsuccessful in helping to relieve her intense distress. She also has major depression, presumed to be secondary to the hypochondriasis.

All three of these patients meet the criteria for the DSM-III-R diagnosis of hypochondriasis. However, their varied presentations demonstrate the clinical heterogeneity within the diagnosis and raise questions about the contribution of comorbid disorders. Mr. A. (Case 1) clearly has OCD as well. Ms. B. (Case 2) is an atypical hypochondriacal individual in that she avoids going to doctors. Ms. C. (Case 3), in addition to hypochondriasis, may have somatization disorder, but the symptoms began after the age of 30 and so she does not meet DSM-III-R criteria. Because of the diverse ways of viewing hypochondriasis, in this chapter we will give a broad overview of the disorder within which the relationship between hypochondriasis and OCD will be examined. History, prevalence, morbidity, comorbidity, and treatment issues will be addressed.

History

Hypochondriasis, which refers literally to a disorder emanating from the "cartilage below the ribs," is an ancient term. Originally it referred to diseases attributed to the digestive organs, the spleen, the bowels, the humours, or animal spirits (Ladee 1966). In the 17th century, Syndenham associated the term with hysteria (Veith 1956). In the mid-19th century, Romberg linked it with heightened nerve sensitivity (Kellner 1986). In the early 20th century, Kraepelin associated hypochondriasis with psychosis (Kraepelin 1919). With the emergence of psychoanalysis, the prevailing understanding emphasized the Freudian view that hypochondriasis arises from a withdrawal of libido from the external world onto internal organs (Freud 1914/1957; Nemiah 1985).

Treatment related directly to the prevailing conceptual framework. In the 18th century, blood letting and purgation were employed to relieve the individual's suffering. In the 20th century, as hypochondriasis came to be seen as a psychological illness, psychotherapy became the main treatment. Until very recently, hypochondriasis was considered to be a disorder with a poor prognosis for which the psychiatrist and internist would need to have much patience and low expectations for improvement (Nemiah 1985).

Definition

Hypochondriasis is defined in the DSM-III-R as a preoccupation with the fear of having, or the belief that one has, a serious disease, based on the person's interpretation of physical signs or sensations as evidence of physical illness. Appropriate physical evaluation does not support the diagnosis of any physical disorder that could account for the physical signs or sensations or the person's unwarranted interpretation of them, and the physical symptoms are not just symptoms of panic attacks. In addition, the fear of having, or the belief that one has, a disease must persist despite medical reassurance, must last at least 6 months, and must not be of delusional intensity.

When the conviction of disease reaches delusional status, the diagnosis of *delusional disorder, somatic subtype* is made. (This disorder was previously known as "monosymptomatic hypochondriacal psychosis".)

Noteworthy in this definition is the emphasis on the fear or belief of "having" a serious illness and a preoccupation with bodily sensations. Irrational fear of illness in general (i.e., simple phobia) or of "getting" seriously ill (i.e., OCD) is not sufficient to make the diagnosis without the individual also having the fear or conviction of "being" ill (Fallon et al. 1991a). Also noteworthy in the definition is the exclusion of those individuals whose hypochondriacal concerns are due primarily to the symptoms associated with panic disorder. This criterion was emphasized in DSM-III-R, but not DSM-III (American Psychiatric Association 1980), as it became clear that patients with panic disorder are often extremely hypochondriacal (Noyes et al. 1986).

Another key aspect of the diagnosis involves excluding patients who may have undetected serious physical illnesses that have atypical presentations, such as systemic lupus erythematosus, Lyme disease, cancer, multiple sclerosis, or thyroid disease. The task of excluding serious physical illnesses becomes extremely difficult when multisystemic, phenomenologically diverse diseases occur for which no definitive serologic tests exist.

Morbidity

Impairment from hypochondriasis ranges from mild to severe. The obsessive focus on illness often may be associated with marked anxiety and depression and may lead to impaired concentration at work and deteriorating interpersonal relationships. In the Columbia University study of DSM-III-R hypochondriacal patients (Fallon et al. 1991b), many subjects experienced substantial difficulty in work and relationships because of their hypochondriacal concerns. For example, one graduate student felt so unable to concentrate because of her illness fears that she felt compelled to take a leave of absence from school. In another case, a man so feared being stricken by dreaded heart disease, despite a normal exam and no history of panic attacks, that he restricted travel in order to be closer to his doctors.

In a recent study of the disability associated with hypochondriasis, patients with DSM-III-R hypochondriasis were found to be significantly more functionally disabled than medically ill patients without hypochondriacal symptoms; this held true on the subscales of basic activities, intermediate activities, social activities, and occupational disability (Barsky et al. 1990b).

Ladee (1966), in a follow-up study of 225 hypochondriacal patients, reported that 7 patients had committed suicide. However, most of these patients also had had a marked depression. The prevalence of suicide among patients with hypochondriasis and no other major Axis I disorder is unknown.

The cost to society may be extensive. Recent research indicates that 6% to 10% of patients who visit a general medical doctor meet the full criteria for hypochondriasis (Kellner et al. 1983–1984; Barsky et al. 1990a). These data suggest that hypochondriacal individuals place a significant burden on the ambulatory health care system.

Prevalence

There are no community prevalence studies of hypochondriasis. However, several lines of evidence indicate that hypochondriasis is one of the more common psychiatric disorders.

Kellner et al. (1983–1984), using the Illness Attitude Questionnaire, assessed hypochondriacal attitudes among 44 patients attending a family practice clinic and 50 randomly chosen employees. The authors found that 9% of the family practice patients and 2% of the employees gave responses indicative of hypochondriasis. A more recent study (Barsky et al. 1990b) conducted in a general medical clinic found that 8.9% of 1,036 patients were rated as hypochondriacal on a screening instrument and that about two-thirds of screen-positive patients received a DSM-III-R diagnosis of hypochondriasis on a semistructured interview. Thus, the point prevalence in this sample was approximately 6%. In another report, Barsky et al. (1990a) estimated the 6-month prevalence of hypochondriasis among patients seen in a medical clinic to be between 4.2% and 6.3%.

In summary, approximately 6% to 9% of patients visiting a physician are hypochondriacal. The prevalence of hypochondriasis in the general population is unknown, though Kellner's data suggest it may be as high as 2%.

Heterogeneity and Descriptive Phenomenology

Recent studies of patients presenting with hypochondriasis based on established diagnostic criteria report a higher proportion of females to males. Using DSM-III criteria, one study of hypochondriacal patients reported that 60% of the 45 patients were female (Kellner 1982). Barsky et al. (1990b) reported that 75.6% of the 41 medical outpatients with DSM-III-R hypochondriasis were female. The average age of the hypochondriacal patients in these two studies varied from 36 years (Kellner 1982) to 57 years (Barsky et al. 1990b). In Kellner's study, the duration of illness ranged from 6 months to 25 years, with a median of 2 years.

The DSM-III-R definition of hypochondriasis gives equal emphasis to fear, conviction, and bodily preoccupation. Any of these may dominate the clinical picture. If fear is dominant but conviction wavers, the patient may avoid going to a doctor—a behavior that calls into question the DSM-III-R criteria that require that a physical examination take place and that medical reassurance be sought.

The *typical hypochondriac* (see Ms. C. in Case 3), one with a high level of illness conviction and somatic preoccupation, is often found in medical outpatient clinics. At times angry, hostile, clinging, narcissistic, and help-rejecting, this patient may confront the physician with a detailed list of multiple physical symptoms and a long history of extensive diagnostic exams. The patient may have been told by many previous doctors that there is no identifiable organic cause for his or her symptoms, but the sensations and fears persist. When one physical disorder is ruled out by careful testing, new symptoms suggestive of another disorder may emerge. Any exploration into life stressors may be viewed suspiciously, confirming the patient's fears that he or she will not be taken seriously. The patient will most likely reject recommendations for a psychiatric consultation because he or she is convinced that the symptoms have an organic origin. Physical symptoms and illness fears are publicly proclaimed. Personality pathology and somatization disorder may be common comorbid conditions.

The *atypical hypochondriac* (see Ms. B. in Case 2) is less often seen in medical clinics, less public in his or her complaints, and less diverse in his or her symptomatology. One or two physical sensations may trigger a fear of a specific illness. This patient may be quite fearful of being seriously ill but avoids going to doctors lest his or her worst fears be confirmed. The patient may secretly check medical books or ask friends for reassurance. These patients may experience their hypochondriacal fears in waves of conviction, at one time being quite certain of being ill, while at other times being fully aware of the irrational nature of their fears. Because of the greater insight of the atypical hypochondriacal patient, he or she may more easily accept the suggestion of a psychiatric consultation. Associated features may include secondary dysthymia or simple phobia.

Research Limitations

Until recently, studies of hypochondriasis consisted largely of a series of retrospective chart reviews of psychiatric patients. Methodological limitations of these studies included the use of retrospective chart review, the lack of structured interviews and diagnostic criteria, and the use of psychiatric patients. More recent studies have been expanded to include patients who visit primary care physicians. This sample may, however, be biased toward those who experience multiple somatic symptoms and who have less insight into the irrationality of their illness fears. Given the problems of comorbidity with other disorders and the heterogeneity of expression within the disorder, descriptive and treatment studies with better methodological design are needed. In addition, genetic and family studies are needed to address the heritability of this disorder.

Comorbidity

A central issue in the literature on hypochondriasis is its relationship to other disorders. Hypochondriacal concerns have been observed in a variety of psychiatric disorders, including major depression (Kellner et al. 1986a), panic disorder (Noyes et al. 1986), simple phobia (Agras et al. 1969), generalized anxiety disorder (Craske et al. 1989), somatization disorder (Barsky et al. 1992), psychosis (Kraepelin 1919; Stenback 1961), personality disorders (Barsky et al. 1990b; Kellner 1983), and OCD (Rasmussen and Tsuang 1986). The extent of comorbidity has led several authors to conclude that hypochondriasis is not an independent disease entity but rather a manifestation of another disorder. Most commonly implicated was a "masked depression" (Ladee 1966; Lesse 1983), although many authors have also been convinced that the underlying problem was primarily an anxiety disorder (Bianchi 1973). The presence of comorbidity may influence treatment outcome if hypochondriasis is simply an overt manifestation of another underlying disorder. Although treatment studies of hypochondriasis have not examined the presence of comorbid diagnoses using standardized interviews, descriptive studies have employed a few strategies to examine further the comorbidity issue.

One approach has been to correlate self-report scores on anxiety, depressive, and hypochondriacal symptoms in mixed samples of patients, such as medical patients and psychiatric patients, and control subjects (Barsky et al. 1986a; Fava et al. 1982; Kellner et al. 1986b). In general, this approach has led to the conclusion that hypochondriacal concerns are associated about equally with anxiety and depression. Self-report symptom questionnaires more recently have been used to compare samples of hypochondriacal and non-hypochondriacal patients. One study revealed that patients with DSM-III hypochondriasis reported more anxiety symptoms than did matched nonhypochondriacal psychiatric outpatients (Kellner et al. 1989). These approaches, while useful in assessing symptoms of anxiety and depression among hypochondriacal patients, do not clarify the role of comorbid disorders.

A second approach has been to distinguish primary from secondary hypochondriasis. Many of the earlier studies of primary and secondary hypochondriasis were done at a time when standardized structured research instruments and clear diagnositic criteria were not available. The studies themselves often differed in their definition of "primary" and "secondary." Whereas some researchers might have used the classification of "primary" for cases in which hypochondriasis dominated the clinical picture, other researchers employed the classification of "primary" only if no other diagnoses could be made (Barsky et al. 1992; Pilowsky 1970).

Two recent studies have examined primary and secondary hypochondriasis. In a study using a nonstructured clinical interview to make DSM-III diagnoses, Kellner (1983) reported that 13 of 36 patients had hypochondriasis alone, while 23 of 36 had concomitant Axis I disorders. The most common additional diagnoses were atypical somatoform disorder and generalized anxiety disorder. In a more recent study of hypochondriasis that used DSM-III-R criteria and a structured interview (the Diagnostic Interview Schedule [DIS]), 79% of the sample of 42 hypochondriacal subjects drawn from a general medicine outpatient clinic had one or more concurrent Axis I disorders, with the greatest overlap noted with depressive and anxiety disorders (Barsky et al. 1992). Noteworthy findings were that hypochondriasis alone seemed relatively uncommon and that, consistent with previous studies, there were very few features that distinguished primary from secondary hypochondriasis, regardless of the definition used.

A third approach has been to examine the frequency of hypo-chondriasis in other DSM-III-R disorders. The results from a variety of studies are summarized below.

Hypochondriasis and Obsessive-Compulsive Disorder

The contamination obsessions of patients with OCD frequently include a fear of germs and of getting ill. At times, these obsessions extend to the fear of being ill. Researchers who specialize in OCD have observed that somatic and health obsessions are common. In a review of 544 patients with OCD, 28% were found to have either somatic obsessions or the fear of getting ill; for 3.1% of the 544 patients, somatic obsessions were the primary manifestation of the OCD (S. A. Rasmussen and W. K. Goodman, unpublished DSM-IV Position Paper, 1989). Somatic obsessions are not, however, neces-sarily the same as hypochondriacal concerns. For example, a patient with OCD might be obsessed with an irregularity on her skin but not fear illness. Or, a patient might be obsessed with a fear of getting asbestosis from asbestos contamination but not actually fear or suspect he had asbestosis.

While no published study has systematically assessed the preva-lence of hypochondriasis among OCD patients, one recent study (Barsky et al. 1992) using a structured diagnostic interview (i.e., the DIS) reported that the lifetime prevalence of OCD among a sample of 42 hypochondriacal patients, although significantly greater than the rate among a control group (9.5% vs. 2.6%, respectively; $P = .04$), was nevertheless low. Unpublished data from the Columbia Univer-sity study (B. A. Fallon, E. Salman, M. R. Liebowitz, unpublished data, 1991) of 21 hypochondriacal patients using the Structured Clinical Interview for DSM-III-R found a higher lifetime prevalence of OCD (33.3%). The different rates may partly be accounted for by sampling differences. Barsky et al.'s sample was drawn from patients in a hospital primary care medical clinic, whereas the Columbia sample consisted largely of patients who were self-referred, responding to an advertisement about hypochondriasis, and willing to come to a psychiatric clinic for evaluation. Patients with greater insight into the irrationality of their fears may be more likely to have OCD than patients with multiple somatic complaints and little insight who repeatedly visit doctors in a medical clinic.

One argument against the notion that hypochondriasis and OCD are similar disorders rests on the widely held belief that patients with OCD recognize their intrusive thoughts as senseless, whereas patients with hypochondriasis consider these thoughts as sensible. However, current ongoing OCD research is challenging this distinction. The fearful thoughts are now observed to fall on a spectrum of certainty, ranging from those obsessions that are recognized as senseless to those that are believed to be true with almost 100% certainty. Some authors have gone so far as to argue that delusions can arise in the course of OCD. For example, Insel and Akiskal (1986) argued that the fears of patients with OCD fall on a spectrum of insight, ranging from obsessional dystonic beliefs to delusional syntonic convictions. This research literature thus is leading to a reexamination of the traditionally held concept that OCD patients recognize their obsessions as unreasonable. For example, a patient with OCD so feared that removing his shirt might cause his skin to come off that he refused to undress himself; after treatment with intravenous clomipramine, he became able to undress without this anxiety and bizarre fear. Degree of conviction, then, cannot be used to distinguish the hypochondriacal patient from the OCD patient.

Obsessive-compulsive disorder has been compared to other disorders as well, based on this concept of a spectrum of insight. For example, Brotman and Jenike (1985) argued that body dysmorphic disorder and monosymptomatic hypochondriacal psychosis are two variants of the same disorder, falling on that hazy spectrum along which overvalued ideas become fixed delusions. Hollander et al. (1989) posed the same reasoning to suggest a continuity between body dysmorphic disorder and delusional disorder, somatic subtype. Indeed, one argument in favor of a relationship between these disorders comes from case reports that suggest responsiveness to serotonin reuptake blockers. For example, Ross et al. (1987) reported on the use of clomipramine to treat a 41-year-old woman who became obsessed with the perception and the conviction that a bad odor emanated from her body. The perception, but not the conviction, was relieved by pimozide, until clomipramine alone was used and both symptoms resolved. Delusional disorder, somatic subtype may actually represent the more severe end of hypochondriasis rather than a disorder that is truly distinct.

Although most patients with hypochondriasis may not have other obsessive or compulsive features, the clinician would do well to ask specifically about the presence of such features given the possibility that hypochondriasis when associated with current or past OCD may be particularly responsive to serotonin reuptake blockers (see section below on treatment).

Hypochondriasis and Depression

Severe hypochondriasis may lead to despair and secondary depressive symptoms (Barsky et al. 1986). Also true, however, is that primary depression may have hypochondriacal features. Several studies have indicated that in the presence of major depression, the treatment of hypochondriasis with antidepressant therapy is often successful (Kellner 1983; Kellner et al. 1986a; Ladee 1966). The argument that hypochondriasis is actually a "masked depression" has been made often (see, e.g., Barsky 1979; Katon et al. 1982a, 1982b; Lesse 1983) and rests on the suggestion that patients in the early stages of depression fixate on the physiological changes occurring in their bodies (e.g., anorexia, insomnia) and become hypochondriacal before they become aware of their depressed feelings.

Hypochondriasis and Panic Disorder

Patients with panic disorder are often quite hypochondriacal. Noyes et al. (1986) reported that ratings on an index of hypochondriasis were as high among 32 patients with panic disorder as those that had been previously reported for patients with hypochondriasis, and that the hypochondriasis ratings significantly decreased after successful treatment of the panic disorder. Until the appearance of DSM-III-R in 1987, the distinction between panic disorder and hypochondriasis was not clear in the diagnostic systems. Prior to DSM-III-R, a diagnosis of hypochondriasis would have been made even if the primary fear related to panic symptoms, such as the fear of having a heart attack in the setting of panic disorder. Given that hypochondriacal concerns are common in the setting of panic attacks, the criteria in DSM-III-R explicitly indicate that a diagnosis of hypochondriasis should not be made if the illness fears are primarily triggered by the symptoms of panic attacks. This ambiguity makes most epidemiologic and treatment studies of hypochondriasis prior to 1987 difficult to interpret.

At times, the distinction between panic disorder with illness fears and hypochondriasis with secondary panic attacks can be hard to make. One clinically useful clue is that hypochondriacal concerns in the setting of panic disorder tend to focus on an acute life-threatening illness such as having a heart attack, whereas primary hypochondriasis tends to be associated with less acute life-threatening disorders such as having leukemia or AIDS.

Hypochondriasis and Somatization Disorder

In both hypochondriasis and somatization disorder, there is the fear or belief that one is sick. However, in the former the cognitive fear or belief is the primary concern, whereas in the latter the multiple unexplained physical symptoms are the primary concern.

The two disorders may often overlap. Hypochondriacal symptoms, for example, were found in 38% of family practice patients with somatization disorder (Oxman and Barrett 1985). Of 42 hypochondriacal patients drawn from a medical outpatient clinic (Barsky et al. 1992), 21% were found to have somatization disorder as compared with 0% of 76 medical patient control subjects ($P = .0001$).

Hypochondriasis and Personality Disorders

Hypochondriasis has been considered by some to represent an immature defense mechanism that serves to ward off anger associated with the need for emotional reliance on others (Perry and Cooper 1989). Although the hypochondriacal defense mechanism may be used by all individuals, it is often found among those with character pathology.

Several attempts have been made to assess the personality patterns of those patients with hypochondriasis. Pilowsky (1970) evaluated the premorbid personality of patients with primary hypochondriasis and reported the following frequencies: obsessional (79% of females; 84% of males); anxiety prone (79% of females; 60% of males); and hypochondriacal (41% of females; 65% of males). Kellner (1983) found that among 36 patients with hypochondriacal neurosis, 12 also had a personality disorder. Among these 12 patients, several personality disorders were represented, and in only one-third of this group was there evidence of a premorbid personality disorder.

The association of personality disorders with DSM-III-R hypochondriasis has not been well studied. In one recent study using a self-report personality inventory (i.e., the Personality Diagnostic Questionnaire), patients with DSM-III-R hypochondriasis were significantly more likely to have a personality diagnosis than were a group of control subjects matched for medical morbidity (Barsky et al. 1990b). Thus, while patients with hypochondriasis may be more likely to have a personality disorder than nonhypochondriacal medical patients, at present the nature of the relationship between personality disorders and hypochondriasis is unclear.

Hypochondriasis and Other Diagnoses

Other disorders in which hypochondriasis has also been commonly reported include generalized anxiety disorder (Craske et al. 1989) and psychotic disorders (Stenback 1961).

Treatment of Hypochondriasis

Until recently, effective treatments for hypochondriasis were lacking and the prognosis was considered poor (Nemiah 1985). Although hypochondriasis has often been referred to as "masked depression," no prospective open or controlled studies have been done to assess the response of patients with hypochondriasis to antidepressant therapy.

The lack of scientific investigation into this disorder can be attributed to several factors, including the hithertofore absence of promising treatments, the difficulty in getting hypochondriacal patients to see a psychiatrist, and the reluctance of these patients to take medication. Although some noncontrolled studies have been done, each has had major methodological flaws. Several researchers attempted to differentiate "primary" from "secondary" hypochondriasis. The studies themselves indicate that those patients with "primary" hypochondriasis often had significant depressive comorbidity and that rarely were those patients with panic disorder distinguished.

Most studies indicate that 40% to 90% of hypochondriacal patients do not respond to psychotherapeutic or psychopharmacological intervention (Kellner 1983; Kenyon 1964; Ladee 1966; Norton 1961; Pilowsky 1968). However, none of these studies used structured interviews to assess comorbidity; standardized treatments; placebo controls; or blind ratings to assess treatment response. Hence, interpretation of the data is difficult. For example, in Pilowsky's (1968) retrospective study, 50% of 66 inpatients with "primary" hypochondriasis improved. However, because half were treated naturalistically with antidepressant somatic therapy, it is likely that many also suffered from a major depression. Kellner's study (1983) looks quite promising in that 64% of 45 patients with DSM-III hypochondriasis were rated as having recovered or been much improved after psychotherapy; however, the treatment was not standardized, the ratings were not done blindly, and no comparison groups were used. Noteworthy was the finding that long duration of illness and presence of a personality disorder were associated with poor outcome. One provocative uncontrolled study reported that 15 of 16 patients with illness phobia were successfully treated using the behavioral techniques of exposure and response prevention (Warwick and Marks 1988). Given that behavior therapy is helpful to patients with OCD (Marks 1981), its efficacy should be formally tested for hypochondriasis as well.

If hypochondriasis is a form of "masked depression," treatment with an antidepressant should be helpful. There are no studies that directly assess this issue; however, reports exist of tricyclics helping to reduce hypochondriacal symptoms in a sample of depressed patients. Kellner et al. (1986a) administered the Illness Attitude Questionnaire (IAQ) to 20 consecutive nonpsychotic inpatients with DSM-III major depression, melancholic type, and to 20 matched control subjects. All patients were treated with amitriptyline and retested on the IAQ 4 weeks later. The results revealed that before treatment, characteristic hypochondriacal responses occurred in over one-third of the melancholic patients, whereas after treatment the number was the same as in control subjects.

Recent work suggests that hypochondriasis may also respond to other pharmacological agents. Bodkin and White (1989) reported using clonazepam successfully to treat a patient who had OCD who also had the hypochondriacal symptom that he feared he had AIDS, despite medical reassurance to the contrary. Kamlana and Gray (1988) reported the successful use of clomipramine to treat a patient who feared he had developed AIDS and that he might transmit the infection to his pregnant wife and unborn baby. Fallon et al. (1991a) reported the successful use of 80 mg of fluoxetine to treat two patients with DSM-III-R hypochondriasis. Viswanathan and Paradis (1991) reported that 40 mg fluoxetine was successful in treating a patient who had a severe fear of having cancer.

Of significance in the recent reports on the pharmacotherapy of hypochondriasis is the successful use of agents with strong serotonergic action. Fluoxetine, a serotonin reuptake blocker, has been shown in controlled and in open series to be effective in the treatment of a variety of psychiatric disorders, including major depression (Rickels et al. 1986), OCD (Liebowitz et al. 1989; Pigott et al. 1990), and panic disorder (Gorman et al. 1987; Schneier et al. 1990). Because of fluoxetine's favorable side-effect profile and its effectiveness in a variety of psychiatric disorders, it has been used in an open treatment study of DSM-III-R hypochondriasis at Columbia University (Fallon et al. 1991b). Our strategy has been to treat hypochondriasis as an OCD-like disorder. OCD has been shown to respond to serotonin reuptake blockers but not to the noradrenergic antidepressant desipramine (Goodman et al. 1990; Leonard et al. 1988). Because at least some cases of hypochondriasis may be pathophysiologically more similar to OCD than to depression, our study used the higher doses of fluoxetine (60–80 mg) found helpful in studies of OCD (Liebowitz et al. 1989) and depression (Altamura et al. 1988), rather than the lower dose (20 mg) that is helpful for depression but often not for OCD (Liebowitz et al. 1989; Rickels et al. 1986). The strategy of treating hypochondriasis as an OCD-like disorder has been used successfully in pharmacological trials in other disorders characterized by marked obsessions and/or compulsions. These disorders include trichotillomania, which responded better to clomipramine than desipramine (Swedo et al. 1989); moral or religious scrupulosity, which benefited from high doses of fluoxetine (Fallon et al. 1990); and body dysmorphic disorder, which also responded to high doses of fluoxetine (Hollander et al. 1989).

A preliminary analysis of the first eight patients who entered our open treatment study of fluoxetine for DSM-III-R hypochondriasis looks promising (Fallon et al. 1991b). Eight patients (mean age 42 ± 13; sex: three males, five females) entered the 12-week study, two of whom dropped out within the first 2 weeks. Patients with major depression were excluded. The dose of fluoxetine was started at 10 or 20 mg and was increased every 2 weeks, as tolerated, to 80 mg/day. Statistically significant decreases between baseline and week 12 were noted in the measures of hypochondriasis (Whiteley Index [Pilowsky 1967]) and anxiety (HAM-A) but not depression (HAM-D). Five of the six patients who completed the study were much improved at 12 weeks (mean fluoxetine dose = 53 ± 24 mg), while only two of the six were much improved at 6 weeks (mean fluoxetine dose = 35 ± 17 mg). One would have expected that if the efficacy of fluoxetine is based on the antiobsessional features, then lower doses of fluoxetine and shorter duration of treatment should not be effective, whereas higher doses and longer treatment would be efficacious. Although the results from our study lend support to this hypothesis, it should be recognized that the greater improvement at 12 weeks may simply reflect the increased length of time on medication. These results must be considered preliminary in that the study was not placebo controlled, the sample was small, and the ratings were not done blindly.

In general, despite the poor design of many of the above treatment studies, the data suggest that hypochondriasis may not be as treatment refractory as previously believed. As in the study of OCD, the emergence of new treatment strategies for hypochondriasis brings hope to a disorder that previously was considered notoriously unresponsive to treatment.

Conclusions

Our purpose in this chapter was to address the question of whether hypochondriasis should be considered a variant of OCD. That question, if addressed alone, would highlight the obsessive and compulsive features found in those patients with hypochondriasis, as well as the treatment studies indicating responsivity to serotonin reuptake blockers. The question, however, is too narrow, as hypochondriasis is seen commonly in a variety of psychiatric disorders other than OCD. The treatment studies all point to the heterogeneity of hypochondriasis, suggesting, for example, that a duration greater than 3 years or a concomitant personality disorder is associated with a poor prognosis, whereas the presence of depression and short duration are associated with good prognosis. Could it be that patients with hypochondriasis of longer than 3 years' duration are more likely to have an OCD-like disorder or primary personality pathology, while those with hypochondriasis of shorter duration are more likely to have a reactive hypochondriasis associated with depression or panic disorder? Hypochondriasis in which there is no other prominent Axis I or Axis II psychiatric disorder indeed may be primarily an obsessional disorder, most like OCD. These questions have important treatment implications; however, at present no conclusions can be drawn.

Further research is needed in many areas: community prevalence studies; genetic and family studies; and placebo-controlled, double-blind pharmacological treatment studies. Studies need to be conducted in several settings in order to compare results among samples drawn from medical outpatient clinics, psychiatric clinics, and the general community. In order to test whether serotonin reuptake blockers have a specific efficacy in the treatment of hypochondriasis, treatment studies might be designed to compare the efficacy of a noradrenergic antidepressant medication such as desipramine with the efficacy of a serotonin reuptake blocker, as has been done in studies of OCD. Neurobiological challenge studies may help to elucidate the role of the serotonergic system in hypochondriasis.

Finally, treatment studies should also examine the efficacy of psychotherapeutic strategies, such as short-term psychodynamic therapy, interpersonal therapy, or behavior therapy.

This review hopefully has served to raise questions and provoke further investigation by indicating the state of our current knowledge and the methodological issues that need to be addressed before hypochondriasis as a primary disorder can be properly understood.

References

Agras S, Sylvester D, Oliveau D: The epidemiology of common fears and phobias. Compr Psychiatry 10:151–156, 1969

Altamura AC, Montgomery SA, Wernicke JF: The evidence for 20 mg a day of fluoxetine as the optimal dose in the treatment of depression. Br J Psychiatry 153 (suppl 3):109–112, 1988

American Psychiatric Association: Diagnostic and Statistical Manual of Mental Disorders, 3rd Edition. Washington, DC, American Psychiatric Association, 1980

American Psychiatric Association: Diagnostic and Statistical Manual of Mental Disorders, 3rd Edition, Revised. Washington, DC, American Psychiatric Association, 1987

Barsky AJ: Patients who amplify bodily symptoms. Ann Intern Med 91:63–70, 1979

Barksy AJ, Wyshak G, Klerman GL: Hypochondriasis: an evaluation of the DSM-III criteria in medical outpatients. Arch Gen Psychiatry 43:493–500, 1986

Barsky AJ, Wyshak G, Klerman GL, et al: The prevalence of hypochondriasis in medical outpatients. Soc Psychiatry Psychiatr Epidemiol 25:89–94, 1990a

Barsky AJ, Wyshak G, Klerman GL: Transient hypochondriasis. Arch Gen Psychiatry 47:746–752, 1990b

Barsky AJ, Wyshak G, Klerman GL: Psychiatric co-morbidity in DSM-III-R hypochondriasis. Arch Gen Psychiatry 49:101–108, 1992

Bianchi GN. Patterns of hypochondriasis: a principal components analysis. Br J Psychiatry 122:541–548, 1973

Bodkin JA, White K: Clonazepam in the treatment of obsessive compulsive disorder associated with panic disorder in one patient. J Clin Psychiatry 50:265–266, 1989

Brotman AW, Jenike MA: Dsymorphophobia and monosymptomatic hypochondriasis (reply to letter of CS Thomas). Am J Psychiatry 142:1121, 1985

Craske MG, Rapee RM, Jackel L, et al: Qualitative dimensions of worry in DSM-III-R generalized anxiety disorder subjects and non-anxious controls. Behav Res Ther 27:397–402, 1989

Fallon BA, Liebowitz MR, Hollander E, et al: The pharmacotherapy of moral or religious scrupulosity. J Clin Psychiatry 51:517–521, 1990

Fallon BA, Javitch JA, Hollander E, et al: Hypochondriasis and obsessive compulsive disorder: overlaps in diagnosis and treatment. J Clin Psychiatry 52:457–460, 1991a

Fallon BA, Liebowitz MR, Schneier F, et al: An open trial of fluoxetine for hypochondriasis, in New Research Program and Abstracts, 144th annual meeting of the American Psychiatric Association, New Orleans, LA, 1991b, NR188, p 93

Fava GA, Pilowsky I, Pierfederici A, et al: Depression and illness behavior in a general hospital: a prevalence study. Psychother Psychosom 38:141–153, 1982

Freud S: On narcissism: an introduction (1914), in the Standard Edition of the Collected Psychological Works of Sigmund Freud, Vol 14. Translated and edited by Strachey J. London, Hogarth, 1957, pp 67–102

Goodman WK, Price LH, Delgado PL, et al: Specificity of serotonin reuptake inhibitors in the treatment of obsessive-compulsive disorder: comparison of fluvoxamine and desipramine. Arch Gen Psychiatry 47:577–585, 1990

Gorman JM, Liebowitz MR, Fyer AJ, et al: An open trial of fluoxetine in the treatment of panic attacks. J Clin Psychopharmacol 7:329–332, 1987

Hollander E, Liebowitz MR, Winchel R, et al: Treatment of body-dysmorphic disorder with serotonin reuptake blockers. Am J Psychiatry 146:768–770, 1989

Insel TR, Akiskal HS: Obsessive-compulsive disorder with psychotic features: a phenomenologic analysis. Am J Psychiatry 143:1527–1533, 1986

Kamlana SH, Gray P: Fear of AIDS (letter). Br J Psychiatry 153:129, 1988

Katon W, Kleinman A, Rosen G: Depression and somatization: a review, Part I. Am J Med 72:127–135, 1982a

Katon W, Kleinman A, Rosen G: Depression and somatization: a review, Part II. Am J Med 72:241–247, 1982b

Kellner R: Psychotherapeutic strategies in hypochondriasis: a clinical study. Am J Psychother 36:146–157, 1982

Kellner R: The prognosis of treated hypochondriasis: a clinical study. Acta Psychiatr Scand 67:69–79, 1983

Kellner R: Somatization and Hypochondriasis. New York, Praeger, 1986

Kellner R, Abbott P, Pathak D, et al: Hypochondriacal beliefs and attitudes in family practice and psychiatric patients. Int J Psychiatry Med 13:127–139, 1983–1984

Kellner R, Fava GA, Lisansky J, et al: Hypochondriacal fears and beliefs in DSM-III melancholia: changes with amitriptyline. J Affective Disord 10:21–26, 1986a

Kellner R, Slocumb JC, Wiggins RJ, et al: The relationship of hypochondriacal fears and beliefs to anxiety and depression. Psychiatr Med 4:15–24, 1986b

Kellner R, Abbott P, Winslow WW, et al: Anxiety, depression, and somatization in DSM-III hypochondriasis. Psychosomatics 30:57–64, 1989

Kenyon FE: Hypochondriasis: a clinical study. Br J Psychiatry 110:478–488, 1964

Kraepelin E: Dementia Praecox and Paraphrenia. Edited by Robertson GM. Chicago, IL, Chicago Medical Book, 1919

Ladee GA: Hypochondriacal Syndromes. New York, Elsevier, 1966

Leonard H, Swedo S, Rapoport JL, et al: Treatment of childhood obsessive compulsive disorder with clomipramine and desmethylimipramine: a double-blind crossover comparison. Psychopharmacol Bull 24:93–95, 1988

Lesse S: The masked depression syndrome—results of a seventeen-year clinical study. Am J Psychother 37:456–475, 1983

Liebowitz MR, Hollander E, Schneier F, et al: Fluoxetine treatment of obsessive-compulsive disorder: an open clinical trial. J Clin Psychopharmacol 9:423–427, 1989

Marks IM: Review of behavioral psychotherapy, I: obsessive-compulsive disorders. Am J Psychiatry 138:584–592, 1981

Nemiah JC: Dissociative disorders (hysterical neurosis, dissociative type), in Comprehensive Textbook of Psychiatry/IV, 4th Edition, Vol 1. Edited by Kaplan HI, Sadock BJ. Baltimore, MD, Williams and Wilkins, 1985, pp 942–957

Norton A: Mental hospitals ins and outs: a survey of patients admitted to a mental hospital in the past 30 years. BMJ 1:528–536, 1961

Noyes R, Reich J, Clancy J, et al: Reduction in hypochondriasis with treatment of panic disorder. Am J Psychiatry 149:631–635, 1986

Oxman TE, Barrett J; Depression and hypochondriasis in family practice patients with somatization disorder. Gen Hosp Psychiatry 7:321–329, 1985

Perry JC, Cooper SH: An empirical study of defense mechanisms, I: clinical interview and life vignette ratings. Arch Gen Psychiatry 46:444–452, 1989

Pigott TA, Pato MT, Bernstein SE, et al: Controlled comparisons of clomipramine and fluoxetine in the treatment of obsessive-compulsive disorder: behavioral and biological results. Arch Gen Psychiatry 47:926–932, 1990

Pilowsky I: Dimensions of hypochondriasis. Br J Psychiatry 113:89–93, 1967

Pilowsky I: The response to treatment in hypochondriacal disorders. Aust N Z J Psychiatry 2:88–94, 1968

Pilowsky I: Primary and secondary hypochondriasis. Acta Psychiatr Scand 46:273–285, 1970

Rasmussen SA, Tsuang MT: Clinical characteristics and family history in DSM-III obsessive-compulsive disorder. Am J Psychiatry 143:317–322, 1986

Rickels K, Amsterdam JD, Avallone MF: Fluoxetine in major depression: a controlled study. Current Therapeutic Research 39:559–563, 1986

Ross CA, Siddiqui AR, Matas M: DSM-III: problems in diagnosis of paranoia and obsessive-compulsive disorder. Can J Psychiatry 32:146–148, 1987

Schneier FR, Liebowitz MR, Davies SO, et al: Fluoxetine in panic disorder. J Clin Psychopharmacol 10:119–121, 1990

Stenback A: Physical disease and hypochondria in psychiatric patients, in Third World Congress of Psychiatry. Montreal, McGill Toronto, 1961, pp 883–887

Swedo SE, Leonard HL, Rapoport JL, et al: A double-blind comparison of clomipramine and desipramine in the treatment of trichotillomania (hair pulling). N Engl J Med 321:497–501, 1989

Veith I: On hysterical and hypochondriacal afflictions. Bull Hist Med 30:233–240, 1956

Viswanathan R, Paradis C: Treatment of cancer phobia with fluoxetine. Am J Psychiatry 148:1090, 1991

Warwick HMC, Marks IM: Behavioural treatment of illness phobia and hypochondriasis: a pilot study of 17 cases. Br J Psychiatry 152:239–241, 1988

Chapter 5

Trichotillomania

Susan E. Swedo, M.D.

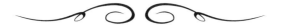

After examining a young man who pulled his hair out in tufts, Hallopeau (1889), a French dermatologist, coined the term *trichotillomania* (from the Greek, meaning "I tear out") to describe the resultant alopecia. It is interesting that Dr. Hallopeau described an adult male with pathological hair pulling, as trichotillomania is more commonly seen in females and usually has its onset in childhood. The term has come to represent the entire syndrome of compulsive hair pulling in which patients are unable to resist impulses to pluck hair from the scalp, eyebrows, eyelashes, or other regions (Krishnan et al. 1985). Patients afflicted with trichotillomania describe an overwhelming urge to pluck out specific hairs; when they do so, the engendered anxiety is momentarily relieved but is quickly replaced by another compulsive urge and even greater anxiety (Swedo and Rapoport 1991).

Trichotillomania has been variously classified as a simple habit disorder (Jillson 1983), as a symptom of psychosis (Oguchi and Miura 1977) or psychodynamic conflict (Greenberg and Sarner 1965), and, currently, as a disorder of impulse control (DSM-III-R 312.39 [American Psychiatric Association 1987]). Before 1980, trichotillomania was included in *Index Medicus* under "Obsessive Compulsive Neurosis," and recent observations have suggested that it might again be classified with obsessive-compulsive disorder (OCD) in a spectrum of disorders having in common pathological grooming compulsions (Demaret 1973; Jenike 1989; Leonard et al. 1991; Swedo 1989; Swedo et al. 1989b).

The question of whether or not trichotillomania is part of a spectrum of obsessive-compulsive–related disorders was first raised by the patients themselves. Following a "20/20" television segment (ABC News, March 1987) concerning OCD, several women telephoned to request treatment for their "hair-pulling compulsion," insisting it was just as disabling and distressing as the checking, hoarding, and hand washing shown on the television program. Their comments sparked a number of ongoing investigations of the similarities and differences between trichotillomania and OCD. In this chapter I will summarize recent studies of the phenomenology, treatment, and neurobiology of trichotillomania. In each instance, consideration will be given to the question: Is trichotillomania an obsessive-compulsive spectrum disorder?

Phenomenology

There are no epidemiologic data available for trichotillomania. Although estimates as high as 2% of the population have been proposed (Azrin and Nunn 1978), the condition has generally been considered to be rare. Gender distribution is also unknown, although clinic samples have been predominantly female (Christenson et al. 1991; Muller 1987). The lack of information about trichotillomania may result from the secrecy of the affected individuals. Hours each day are spent camouflaging the condition, and in several cases the patient said her spouse was unaware of her baldness because she was never without a wig. Many of the patients reported that they thought they were the only one afflicted with this condition and had not sought therapy because of embarrassment or fear of being thought mentally ill. This secrecy is not unlike that seen with OCD several years ago (Swedo et al. 1989d) and may reflect a similar "rational" irrationality:

trichotillomanic patients know the hair pulling is "crazy" and yet they cannot stop.

Since April of 1987, 45 adolescents and adults with trichotillomania have participated in clinical studies at the Child Psychiatry Branch of the National Institute of Mental Health (NIMH). The subjects were self-referred in response to television and magazine publicity and to advertisements placed in a local newsletter and in the Obsessive Compulsive Disorder Foundation newsletter, seeking patients for drug treatment studies of hair pulling.

Inclusionary criteria for the studies were repetitive, compulsive pulling out of the hair considered unreasonable and undesirable by the subject, and observable hair loss. The symptoms had to have been present for at least 1 year, meet DSM-III-R (312.39) diagnostic criteria, and be of sufficient severity to interfere with the patient's daily life because of embarrassment about personal appearance and/or time lost to hair-pulling episodes. Concomitant OCD was an exclusionary criterion, as were physical illness, mental retardation, primary affective disorder, psychosis, evidence of neurological damage, and uncooperativeness with study procedures. As in previous studies, prior history of depression or anxiety disorder, or secondary depression, were not reasons for exclusion from the study. Of the applicants to the study, two were excluded for concomitant OCD, one for psychosis, and two for primary affective disorder. In addition, two subjects exhibited depressive symptoms at screening, and entry into the study was delayed until the symptoms abated. Five potential subjects chose not to participate after the study was explained to them.

The mean (± SD) age of the 30 females and 14 males at presentation was 30.2 (± 10.5) years, the mean age at onset of hair pulling was 11.5 (± 6.1) years, and the mean duration of the condition was 18.6 (± 11.1) years. As documented for OCD (Rasmussen and Eisen 1990; Swedo et al. 1989b), the mean age at presentation, age at onset, and duration of illness of the males were less than for the females, despite similar recruiting efforts. The onset of hair pulling occurred slightly before puberty in most male cases and during early adolescence in most females. The majority of patients pulled scalp hair, although eyebrows and eyelashes were also frequently pulled. Previous treatments included a variety of behavior therapy techniques, hypnosis, psychotherapy, and pharmacotherapy with antidepressant, anxiolytic, and antipsychotic agents.

Clinical Presentation

In severe cases, trichotillomanic patients spend several hours each day pulling their hair or thinking about pulling. These patients exhibit large, irregularly shaped bald areas interspersed with few, short regrowing hairs. Frequently, hairs at the occiput and base of the head are spared (Dawber 1985), resulting in the tonsural pattern of baldness typifying severe trichotillomania. Less severely affected patients may have only small areas of baldness or imperceptible thinning over the entire head. In addition, eyelashes, eyebrows, body hair, and pubic hair may be pulled.

Just as OCD patients describe an overwhelming anxiety accompanying a compulsive urge that is relieved temporarily by performing the ritual, trichotillomanic patients describe an irresistible impulse and concomitant anxiety that cause them to pull out a specific hair. Frequently, the chosen hair is identified as different from the others (e.g., too kinky/straight, brittle/supple, etc.), and its removal is necessary in order to make the hair feel "just right." Despite a definite sense of knowing which one hair is sought, many hairs are pulled in order to get just the right one. Tweezers might be utilized to get the entire hair out, but the patients rarely report associated pain. Some patients compulsively pick at the scalp, in addition to pulling the hair, resulting in numerous painful traumatic lesions. After plucking the hair, the trichotillomanic patient frequently will stroke it against the cheek and/or lips and might eat the root or entire hair. Some patients have elaborate rituals surrounding the hair pulling, while others pluck one after another in rapid succession, with little or no accompanying cognition. Thus, a patient may spend 2 hours pulling 20–25 hairs, or he or she may pull the same number in a few minutes.

In contrast to patients with OCD compulsions, trichotillomanic patients do not pull their hair in response to an obsessive thought, such as harm coming to self or loved ones, but only because of an irresistible urge and accompanying anxiety. In addition, OCD patients have compulsions that are considered to be ego-dystonic, whereas many trichotillomanic patients report the hair pulling as being pleasurable. Also unlike patients with OCD, whose symptoms change over time (e.g., counting evolves into repeating, which is then replaced by washing), trichotillomanic patients only pull their hair— they do not substitute other compulsive rituals for this behavior.

Clinical Assessment

Severity of trichotillomania was rated with three measures, described elsewhere in detail (Swedo et al. 1989b) and summarized below:

1. The Trichotillomania Symptom Severity Scale (range of scores: 0 to 20), consisting of five items evaluating 1) average time spent pulling each day, 2) average time spent pulling on prior day, 3) amount of resistance against the hair-pulling urge, 4) degree of subjective distress, and 5) interference with daily activities.
2. The Trichotillomania Impairment Scale (range of scores: 0 to 10): Assessment of overall impairment resulting from the trichotillomania, in which 0 represents total lack of symptoms and 10 indicates severe impairment (majority of time each day spent pulling or resisting the urge to pull out the hair, and large bald patches or total denudation evident).
3. Physician's Rating of Clinical Progress (range or scores: 0 to 20): Assessment of clinical change, in which 0 represents a total "cure," 10 the pretreatment baseline, and 20 the worst possible or total incapacitation secondary to the trichotillomania.

The Schedule for Affective Disorders and Schizophrenia—Lifetime Version (SADS-L) (Spitzer and Endicott 1978) and the Structured Interview for Personality Disorders (SID-P) (Stangl et al. 1985) were administered to the adult subjects, and the Diagnostic Interview for Children and Adolescents (DICA) (Welner et al. 1987) to subjects aged 6 to 18 years, in order to identify associated psychopathology. The family studies also utilized these structured interviews.

Associated Psychopathology

The SADS-L and the SID-P were administered to 30 adult trichotillomanic subjects (22 females and 8 males), and the DICA to those
subjects 9 to 18 years of age (2 females and 5 males). This study, the
first systematic study of comorbidity of trichotillomania, revealed
associated Axis I psychopathology in 29 (78%) and Axis II personality
disorders in 14 (38%) of the 37 subjects. Fifteen patients met criteria
for unipolar depression, 12 for generalized anxiety disorder, 2 for
bipolar disorder, 6 for substance abuse, and 2 for panic disorder. Axis
II disorders included histrionic ($n = 10$), borderline ($n = 7$) and
passive-aggressive ($n = 7$) personality disorders. Despite excluding
patients from the study who had concomitant OCD, 5 patients had a
past history of obsessive-compulsive behaviors, although in some
cases these behaviors did not meet severity criteria for the diagnosis
of OCD. (For example, a 16-year-old female recalled having had
counting and repeating rituals between the ages of 8 and 10, which
disappeared when her hair pulling started; a 32-year-old male had
had washing rituals before the onset of his trichotillomania.) In OCD,
comorbidity also is reported frequently (50%–75% of patients) (reviewed by Rasmussen and Eisen 1990); as is seen in trichotillomania,
the most common diagnoses associated with OCD are affective
disorder and anxiety disorders (Rasmussen and Eisen 1990; Swedo
et al. 1989d).

Family Studies

In-person interviews were conducted with all first-degree relatives
(i.e., parents, siblings, and offspring) of 28 consecutive trichotillomanic patients in order to determine whether there was an increased
rate of trichotillomania, OCD, or other psychopathology among the
family members. Sixty-five first-degree relatives of 16 female trichotillomanic probands and 41 parents and siblings of 12 male trichotillomanic probands were interviewed with the SADS-L or the DICA
(depending on the subject's age) and a brief questionnaire designed
to elicit a history of trichotillomania (M. C. Lenane, S. E. Swedo, H.
L. Leonard, et al., unpublished questionnaire, 1989). Similar informa-

tion was obtained from a group of control subjects and from a contrast group of parents of probands with conduct disorder. All interviews were scored by a rater blind to proband diagnosis.

One parent, three siblings, and one offspring received a diagnosis of trichotillomania. None of the 65 subjects in the age-matched contrast group received this diagnosis. Although the prevalence of trichotillomania is unknown, in comparison with the normal control subjects, the relatives of the trichotillomanic probands exhibited a slight, although not statistically significant, increase in hair pulling.

Two parents, two siblings, and one offspring met criteria for a lifetime diagnosis of OCD (5% of relatives). Only one (1.5%) of the parents of conduct-disorder probands met criteria for OCD; however, the 5% prevalence of OCD among the first-degree relatives of the trichotillomanic probands is not significantly increased over that of the contrast group (Lenane et al. 1990, in press).

In summary, the hair pulling of trichotillomania appears to be quite phenomenologically similar to the compulsive rituals of OCD. Trichotillomania differs from OCD by the lack of symptom progression and the absence of concomitant obsessive thoughts. The presence of OCD among 5% of first-degree relatives of trichotillomanic probands may suggest a genetic association between the two disorders, but further investigations are required.

Pediatric Trichotillomania

Trichotillomania that has its onset in infancy and early childhood is considered separately here because it may be a different disorder from that which presents during adolescence and young adulthood. Early-onset trichotillomania has been described as a habit disorder (Jillson 1983; Price 1978) analogous to nail biting (Oguchi and Miura 1977), and as a symptom of an impaired mother-child relationship (Aleksandrowicz and Mares 1978; Mannino and Delgado 1969, among others). It is unclear from published reports whether hair pulling with onset before 5 years of age constitutes the same disorder as that which presents during adolescence and young adulthood; the literature is dichotomous, with little overlap between the two age groups. (For a review of pediatric trichotillomania, see, for example, Delgado and Mannino 1969.) Some differences are apparent; for example, Muller (1987) reported that 62% of preschool-age trichotillomanic children were males versus 30% males for other age groups. In addition, unlike the chronic, debilitating condition that affects adolescents and young adults, early-onset trichotillomania is reported to be benign and self-limited (Stroud 1983). Longitudinal reports are not available, but it appears that early-onset trichotillomania may be "outgrown" and that it does not continue into adolescence or adulthood (Oranje et al. 1986). Our sample of older patients seems to support this, as no patient is reported to have begun pulling before the age of 5.

We have evaluated 10 infants and children (7 females and 3 males) with trichotillomania. For the study of early-onset trichotillomania, all children 7 years of age or less who had alopecia secondary to observed hair pulling and who had begun pulling before age 5 were accepted. These children are participating in an ongoing, naturalistic, longitudinal study that will be used to define the natural history and prognosis of early-onset trichotillomania. The children begin pulling at a very young age and pull scalp hair almost exclusively (9 scalp, 2 eyebrows/eyelashes). The children typically present at age 4 with a 22-month history of pulling their scalp hair, particularly during stressful periods and after being put down for sleep. Occasionally, the parents will report that the child pulls during his or her sleep, but typically it is only while the child is awake. If prevented from pulling, the child may desist but will return to pulling when intervention stops. Some children exhibit anger or anxiety when prevented, whereas others do not seem to mind the parental intervention. The parents report that there is no apparent anxiety preceding the pulling, but the children are too young to verify this information.

Unlike their adult counterparts, the children have a clinical course that is frequently episodic, with periods of complete remission occurring 2–3 times each year. Interestingly, the periods of relapse are most frequently seen in October or November, and in February. This raises the question of an environmental event releasing the hair pulling. This author has speculated that the children might have an underlying genetic susceptibility that is expressed in response to an autoimmune reaction, triggered by a bacterial or viral infection (such as streptococcal or varicella [chickenpox] infections) (Swedo 1989; Swedo et al. 1989c, 1991b). Serial blood samples are being obtained from the children during quiescent periods and periods of relapse to determine titers of antistreptococcal antibodies and antineuronal antibodies (Husby et al. 1976; Swedo et al. 1989c).

Structured interviews (SADS-L and DICA) have been administered to 24 first-degree relatives of 9 early-onset trichotillomanic children. There was only one parent with trichotillomania (5%) among these first-degree relatives, and no OCD has been seen in parents or siblings of these children to date. It is interesting, however, that three of the mothers had had an anxiety disorder during childhood. A larger sample is needed before we can draw any conclusions about familiality in early-onset trichotillomania.

Treatment

Perhaps the most compelling evidence for inclusion of trichotillomania within a spectrum of obsessive-compulsive–related disorders comes from the demonstrated superiority of clomipramine, an anti-obsessional drug (Leonard et al. 1989b; Mavissakalian et al. 1985; Thorén et al. 1980), over desipramine, a standard tricyclic antidepressant with little antiobsessional efficacy (Insel et al. 1983; Leonard et al. 1989b), for the treatment of trichotillomania (Swedo et al. 1989b). We have previously reported the results of 14 females with trichotillomania treated in a double-blind crossover comparison study of clomipramine versus desipramine (Swedo et al. 1989b), but have now extended the sample to include a total of 22 subjects (19 females, 3 males).

The methods have been described elsewhere (see Swedo et al. 1989). In brief, a 2-week, single-blind placebo phase preceded the active-treatment comparison, and any patient with greater than 20% reduction in symptomatology during this phase was excluded from data analysis. The active-treatment comparison consisted of two consecutive 5-week periods of treatment with either clomipramine or desipramine, administered in a double-blind manner in a randomly assigned order. Patients were started on 25 or 50 mg/day and advanced as tolerated to a maximum of 3 mg/kg of body weight/day (250 mg/day). At the end of the first active-treatment phase, the dose of the first drug was tapered over the first 5 to 7 days of the second phase while the second drug was being given in gradually increasing doses.

The patients were interviewed weekly to evaluate the symptoms of trichotillomania, depression, and anxiety, and to identify any side effects of the medication. Trichotillomania severity was rated with the three measures described earlier in this chapter.

The results for the 22 patients are shown in Table 5–1. For each of the trichotillomania symptom ratings, clomipramine was strikingly superior to desipramine in reducing symptom severity. As can be seen in the table, anxiety and depression also were reduced more by clomipramine than by desipramine, although neither reduction was clinically significant. Side effects did not differ significantly between clomipramine and desipramine, with both drugs being tolerated fairly well.

Baseline trichotillomania symptom severity scale scores were negatively correlated with improvement (Pearson correlation coefficients: -0.4 and -0.5 [$P = .04$ and $.02$, respectively] for scores on the Trichotillomania Symptom Severity Scale and Trichotillomania Impairment Scale, respectively), so that more symptomatic patients showed less improvement. (The expression of the change measures as percent improvement may have affected these correlations.) In addition, comorbidity affected treatment outcome. Patients with a concomitant anxiety disorder or with borderline personality disorder were less likely to respond to clomipramine therapy. Based on t tests comparing mean percent change on the Trichotillomania Impairment Scale, significant differences in response were seen for patients with anxiety disorders (11 patients, mean = 18.7% improvement) and those without comorbid anxiety disorders (11 patients, mean = 48.0%) ($t = 2.28$, $P = .03$), and for patients with (5 patients, mean = 6.7%) and without (17 patients, mean = 41.2%) borderline personality disorder ($t = 2.24$, $P = .03$). The borderline patients showed very little change on the Trichotillomania Symptom Severity Scale (mean change = 7.5% vs. 49.1% for nonborderline patients; $t = 2.70$, $P = .01$).

Table 5–1. Clinical ratings during clomipramine and desipramine treatment of trichotillomania

Scale	Baseline	Placebo	Desipramine	Clomipramine	Clomipramine vs. Desipramine	
					t	p
Severity of symptoms	16.3 ± 3.9	15.4 ± 5.0	13.6 ± 5.8	10.4 ± 7.2	2.19	.04
Trichotillomania impairment	6.8 ± 1.7	6.8 ± 1.6	6.1 ± 2.2	4.6 ± 2.6	2.81	.01
Clinical progress	10.0 ± 0	10.0 ± 1.0	8.5 ± 3.1	5.2 ± 3.7	3.67	.01
Anxiety	4.0 ± 1.6	3.5 ± 1.3	2.8 ± 1.3	2.1 ± 1.2	2.19	.04
Depression	2.6 ± 1.4	2.5 ± 1.2	2.5 ± 1.5	1.6 ± 1.1	3.10	.006

Note. All comparisons between the drugs were made by two-tailed, paired t test. The ratings shown are those made after 5 weeks of treatment with each of the two drugs. For description of the various scales, see section on methods in text.

Following our report of clomipramine's efficacy, another serotonin reuptake blocker, fluoxetine, was reported to be effective in several open trials (Benarroche 1990; Stanley et al. 1990; Winchel et al. 1989). The effectiveness of fluoxetine and clomipramine, but not desipramine, in the treatment of trichotillomania suggests that serotonin reuptake blockade may mediate the antitrichotillomanic effect.

Long-Term Outcome

Because anecdotal experience had suggested that the effectiveness of serotonin reuptake blocking drugs may wane with time, long-term outcome of the first 16 consecutive participants in the clomipramine-desipramine treatment study was assessed at 2-year follow-up. Fourteen of these women were interviewed in person and two by telephone, utilizing the three trichotillomania rating scales and a clinical interview for interval history. Associated psychopathology remained common. In addition, one woman had manifest symptoms of bipolar disorder since completion of the study, and another had suffered a major depressive episode during the intervening 2 years.

When considered as a group, there was still significant (40%) improvement in severity of trichotillomania from the pretreatment baseline, although individual response varied widely. Four women (25%) had marked (80%–100%) improvement from baseline. All were currently taking either clomipramine or fluoxetine, and one had had behavior therapy. Three women had moderate (40%–75%) improvement and two mild (10%–30%) improvement, but seven remained unchanged. In some cases, patients had had a dramatic reduction in hair-pulling symptoms during the first few months of therapy and then relapsed, despite continued pharmacotherapy.

Behavioral treatment had been recommended to all patients but was obtained by only five. In no case was behavior therapy effective if the patient had not responded (at least partially) to drug treatment. All five patients had found behavior therapy helpful, although only one obtained a complete remission during this therapy. The patient who achieved complete remission was treated with a combination of exposure and response prevention (Mansueto and Goldfinger 1990) and habit reversal (Azrin et al. 1980).

Neurobiology

Patients with OCD had previously been shown to perform more poorly on the Street Map Test (Money et al. 1965) and the Stylus Maze Test (Milner 1965) than normal control subjects (Behar et al. 1984; Cox et al. 1989; Head et al. 1989). These neuropsychological tests are felt to reflect dysfunction in the caudate and/or frontal, and frontal-parietal regions, respectively. The Street Map and Stylus Maze were administered to 21 female patients with severe trichotillomania, and the results were compared with those of 12 OCD patients, 17 patients with other anxiety disorders, and 16 normal control subjects (Rettew et al. 1991). There were no significant group differences in performance on the Street Map Test. The trichotillomania group made significantly more errors on the Stylus Maze than did the normal control group, and, further, the number of errors committed was positively correlated with baseline trichotillomania symptom severity and negatively correlated with improvement following clomipramine therapy. Because the trichotillomanic patients performed more like the OCD subjects than like the normal control subjects or patients with anxiety disorders, these results were felt to reflect neuropsychological similarities between the trichotillomanic and OCD patients.

Several studies have utilized positron-emission tomography (PET) to measure regional cerebral glucose metabolism in OCD patients. These studies have shown hypermetabolism of the orbital frontal region in comparison with normal control subjects (Baxter et al. 1987, 1988; Nordahl et al. 1989; Swedo et al. 1989e). Although results vary by center and scanning technique, the caudate nuclei and prefrontal and anterior cingulate regions also appear to be hypermetabolic in OCD. This regional hypermetabolism appears to be related to symptom severity and treatment response, as two groups of researchers have reported normalization following pharmacotherapy (Baxter et al. 1987; Benkelfat et al. 1990). In addition, baseline anterior cingulate and orbital frontal metabolism was inversely related to response to clomipramine therapy in a group of childhood-onset OCD patients such that nonresponders had greater hypermetabolism than did responders (Swedo et al. 1989e).

Ten adult females with trichotillomania and 20 age-matched

female control subjects were scanned in the resting state using PET and ^{18}F-labeled fluorodeoxyglucose (Swedo et al. 1991a). The trichotillomanic patients demonstrated striking and significant increases in global (mean gray matter) metabolism, as well as higher normalized right superior parietal and right and left cerebellar glucose metabolic rates, than did the normal control subjects. None of these regions had been hypermetabolic in the OCD subjects, although the cerebellar region had not usually been examined previously.

Orbital frontal and anterior cingulate hypermetabolism was negatively correlated with improvement following clomipramine therapy in the trichotillomanic patients, as was true for the childhood-onset OCD subjects scanned under identical conditions (Swedo et al. 1989e, 1991a). Because clomipramine nonresponders had greater anterior cingulate and orbital frontal hypermetabolism than did responders, one might speculate that the hypermetabolism represents compensatory efforts to overcome pathological rituals initiated elsewhere. Although it is premature to assign meaning to these preliminary findings, it is intriguing that two disorders, trichotillomania and OCD, with similar clinical response to specific drug therapy, demonstrated similar baseline regional glucose metabolic patterns predicting response to clomipramine treatment. This association between drug response and baseline patterns of glucose metabolism may be useful in pinpointing regional involvement in other disorders as well.

In summary, trichotillomanic and OCD patients had similar performance on the Street Map Test, and similar negative associations between regional hypermetabolism and response to clomipramine therapy, but different baseline patterns of PET glucose metabolism. Additional neurobiological investigations, including anatomic and functional investigations, are indicated.

Conclusions

Trichotillomania is a neglected neuropsychiatric disorder that has only recently received research attention. Based on clinical data, it appears far more common than previously believed. Like OCD (and tics), the behavior is recognized as senseless and undesirable but is performed in response to increasing anxiety, with resultant tension relief. The condition may be episodic but is usually chronic and difficult to treat. Both the comorbidity and the phenomenology of trichotillomania extend the concept of OCD to a spectrum of inappropriately released, excessive grooming behaviors. The most compelling evidence for placing trichotillomania within the spectrum of obsessive-compulsive–related disorders remains the selective effectiveness of clomipramine, a documented antiobsessional compound, for the treatment of trichotillomania. Although the discovery of clomipramine's effectiveness has provided relief to some trichotillomanic patients, further work is indicated to find regimens that will provide long-term suppression of symptoms. Ongoing investigations of early-onset trichotillomania may reveal etiologic triggers to this puzzling disorder, while studies that examine the similarities and differences between trichotillomania and OCD may help define the neurobiology of OCD, and possibly of other atypical impulse control disorders.

References

Aleksandrowicz MK, Mares AJ: Trichotillomania and trichobezoar in an infant: psychological factors underlying this symptom. Journal of the American Academy of Child Psychiatry 17:533–539, 1978

American Psychiatric Association: Diagnostic and Statistical Manual of Mental Disorders, 3rd Edition, Revised. Washington, DC, American Psychiatric Association, 1987

Azrin NH, Nunn RG: Habit Control in a Day. New York, Simon & Schuster, 1978

Azrin NH, Nunn RG, Frantz SE: Treatment of hairpulling (trichotillomania): a comparative study of habit reversal and negative practice training. J Behav Ther Exp Psychiatry 11:13–20, 1980

Baxter LR Jr, Phelps ME, Mazziotta JC, et al: Local cerebral glucose metabolic rates in obsessive-compulsive disorder: a comparison with rates in unipolar depression and in normal controls. Arch Gen Psychiatry 44:211–218, 1987

Baxter LR Jr, Schwartz JM, Mazziotta JC, et al: Cerebral glucose metabolic rates in nondepressed patients with obsessive-compulsive disorder. Am J Psychiatry 145:1560–1563, 1988

Behar D, Rapoport JL, Berg CJ: Computerized tomography and neuropsychological test measures in adolescents with obsessive-compulsive disorder. Am J Psychiatry 141:363–369, 1984

Benarroche CL: Trichotillomania symptoms and fluoxetine response, in New Research Program and Abstracts, 143rd annual meeting of the American Psychiatric Association, New York, NY, May 1990, NR327, p 173

Benkelfat C, Nordahl TE, Semple WE, et al: Local cerebral glucose metabolic rates in obsessive-compulsive disorder: patients treated with clomipramine. Arch Gen Psychiatry 47:840–848, 1990

Christenson GA, Mackenzie TB, Mitchell JE: Characteristics of 60 adult chronic hair pullers. Am J Psychiatry 148:365–370, 1991

Cox CS, Fedio P, Rapoport JL: Neuropsychological testing of obsessive-compulsive adults, in Obsessive-Compulsive Disorder in Children and Adolescents. Edited by Rapoport JL. Washington, DC, American Psychiatric Press, 1989, pp 73–85

Dawber R: Self-induced hair loss. Seminars in Dermatology 4:53–57, 1985

Delgado RA, Mannino FV: Some observations on trichotillomania in children. Journal of the American Academy of Child Psychiatry 8:229–246, 1969

Demaret A: Onychophagia, trichotillomania and grooming. Ann Med Psychol (Paris) 1:235–242, 1973

Greenberg HR, Sarner CA: Trichotillomania: symptom and syndrome. Arch Gen Psychiatry 12:482–489, 1965

Hallopeau M: Alopecie par grottage (trichomanie ou trichotillomanie). Ann Dermatol Venereol 10:440–441, 1889

Head D, Bolton D, Hymas N: Deficit in cognitive shifting ability in patients with obsessive-compulsive disorder. Biol Psychiatry 25:929–937, 1989

Husby G, vandeRyn I, Zabriskie JB, et al: Antibodies reacting with cytoplasm of subthalamic and caudate nuclei neurons in chorea and rheumatic fever. J Exp Med 144:1094–1110, 1976

Insel TR, Murphy DL, Cohen RM, et al: Obsessive-compulsive disorder: a double-blind trial of clomipramine and clorgyline. Arch Gen Psychiatry 40:605–612, 1983

Jillson OT: Alopecia, II: trichotillomania (trichotillohabitus). Cutis 31:383–389, 1983

Krishnan KRR, Davidson JRT, Guajardo C: Trichotillomania—a review. Compr Psychiatry 26:123–128, 1985

Lenane MC, Swedo SE, Leonard H, et al: Psychiatric disorders in first degree relatives of children and adolescents with obsessive-compulsive disorder. J Am Acad Child Adolesc Psychiatry 29:407–412, 1990

Lenane MC, Swedo SE, Rapoport JL, et al: Increased rates of obsessive-compulsive disorder in first-degree relatives of patients with trichotillomania. J Child Psychol Psychiatry (in press)

Leonard HL, Swedo SE, Rapoport JL, et al: Treatment of obsessive-compulsive disorder with clomipramine and desipramine in children and adolescents: a double-blind crossover comparison. Arch Gen Psychiatry 46:1088–1092, 1989b

Leonard HL, Lenane M, Swedo SE, et al: A double-blind comparison of clomipramine and desipramine treatment of severe onychophagia (nail-biting). Arch Gen Psychiatry 48:821–827, 1991

Mannino FV, Delgado RA: Trichotillomania in children: a review. Am J Psychiatry 126:505–511, 1969

Mansueto C, Goldfinger RI: Group treatment of trichotillomania with multi-system habit competition training. Symposium presented at the annual meeting of the Association for the Advancement of Behavior Therapy, San Francisco, CA, November 1990

Mavissakalian M, Turner SM, Michelson L, et al: Tricyclic antidepressants in obsessive-compulsive disorder: antiobsessional or antidepressant agents? II. Am J Psychiatry 142:572–576, 1985

Milner B: Visually-guided maze learning in man: effects of bilateral hippocampal, bilateral frontal and unilateral cerebral lesions. Neuropsychologia 3:317–338, 1965

Money J, Alexander D, Walker HT: A Standardized Road Map Test of Direction Sense. Baltimore, MD, Johns Hopkins University Press, 1965

Muller SA: Trichotillomania. Dermatol Clin 5:595–601, 1987

Nordahl TE, Benkelfat C, Semple WE, et al: Cerebral glucose metabolic rates in obsessive-compulsive disorder. Neuropsychopharmacology 2:23–28, 1989

Oguchi T, Miura S: Trichotillomania: its psychopathological aspect. Compr Psychiatry 18:177–182, 1977

Oranje AP, Peereboom-Wynia JDR, De Raeymaecker DMJ: Trichotillomania in childhood. J Am Acad Dermatol 15:614–619, 1986

Price VH: Disorders of the hair in children. Pediatr Clin North Am 25:305–320, 1978

Rasmussen SA, Eisen JL: Epidemiology and clinical features of obsessive-compulsive disorder, in Obsessive-Compulsive Disorders: Theory and Management. Edited by Jenike MA, Baer L, Minichiello WE. Chicago, IL, Year Book Medical, 1990, pp 10–27

Rettew DC, Cheslow DL, Rapoport JL, et al: Neuropsychological test performance in trichotillomania: a further link with obsessive-compulsive disorder. Journal of Anxiety Disorders 5:225–235, 1991

Spitzer R, Endicott J: Schedule for Affective Disorders and Schizophrenia, 3rd Edition. Biometrics Research Division, New York State Psychiatric Institute, New York, 1978

Stangl D, Pfohl B, Zimmerman M, et al: A structured interview for the DSM-III personality disorders: a preliminary report. Arch Gen Psychiatry 42:591–596, 1985

Stanley MA, Bowers TC, Swann AC: Trichotillomania and obsessive compulsive disorder, in New Research Program and Abstracts, 143rd annual meeting of the American Psychiatric Association, New York, NY, May 1990, NR292, p 158

Stroud JD: Hair loss in children. Pediatr Clin North Am 30:641–657, 1983

Swedo SE: Rituals and releasers: an ethological model of obsessive-compulsive disorder, in Obsessive-Compulsive Disorder in Children and Adolescents. Edited by Rapoport JL. Washington DC, American Psychiatric Press, 1989, pp 269–288

Swedo SE, Rapoport JL: Annotation: trichotillomania. J Child Psychol Psychiatry 32:401–409, 1991

Swedo SE, Kruesi MJP, Leonard HL, et al: Lack of seasonal variation in pediatric lumbar cerebrospinal fluid neurotransmitter metabolite concentrations. Acta Psychiatr Scand 80:644–649, 1989a

Swedo SE, Leonard HL, Rapoport JL, et al: A double-blind comparison of clomipramine and desipramine in the treatment of trichotillomania (hair pulling). N Engl J Med 321:497–501, 1989b

Swedo SE, Rapoport JL, Cheslow DL, et al: High prevalence of obsessive-compulsive symptoms in patients with Sydenham's chorea. Am J Psychiatry 146:246–249, 1989c

Swedo SE, Rapoport JL, Leonard H, et al: Obsessive-compulsive disorder in children and adolescents: clinical phenomenology of 70 consecutive cases. Arch Gen Psychiatry 46:335–341, 1989d

Swedo SE, Schapiro MB, Grady CL, et al: Cerebral glucose metabolism in childhood-onset obsessive-compulsive disorder. Arch Gen Psychiatry 46:518–523, 1989e

Swedo SE, Grady CL, Leonard HL, et al: Regional cerebral glucose metabolism of women with trichotillomania. Arch Gen Psychiatry 48:828–833, 1991a

Swedo SE, Kilpatrick K, Schapiro M, et al: Antineuronal antibodies (AnA) in Sydenham's chorea (SC) and obsessive-compulsive disorder (OCD). Pediatr Res 29(4:2): 364A, 1991b, no 2166

Thorén P, Åsberg M, Cronholm B, et al: Clomipramine treatment of obsessive-compulsive disorder, I: a controlled clinical trial. Arch Gen Psychiatry 37:1281–1285, 1980

Welner Z, Reich W, Herjanic B, et al: Reliability, validity and parent-child agreement studies of the Diagnostic Interview for Children and Adolescents (DICA). J Am Acad Child Adolesc Psychiatry 26:649–653, 1987

Winchel R, Stanley B, Guido J, et al: An open trial of fluoxetine for trichotillomania (hairpulling). Poster presented at the 28th annual meeting of the American College of Neuropsychopharmacology, Maui, HI, December 1989

Chapter 6

Tourette's Syndrome

James F. Leckman, M.D.

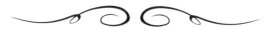

Tourette's syndrome (TS) is a lifelong disorder of unknown etiology. The range of symptoms encountered in this disorder includes motor and phonic tics (sudden repetitive movements, gestures or utterances that typically mimic some aspect of the normal behavioral repertoire) and, in a sizeable proportion of cases, obsessions and compulsions (sudden repetitive thoughts, images, or urges to act that are intrusive and difficult to resist). Less well appreciated are the sensorimotor phenomena that frequently accompany tics and obsessive-compulsive behaviors. These experiences include premonitory feelings or urges that are relieved with the performance of the

Aspects of this research were supported in part by the National Institutes of Health (Grants RR-00125, MH-30929, HD-03008, and MH-44843), the Gateposts Foundation, the Tourette Syndrome Association, the Leon Lowenstein Foundation, and the John Merck Fund. Portions of this chapter are based in part on a chapter by J. F. Leckman and D. J. Cohen in the book *Child and Adolescent Psychiatry: A Comprehensive Textbook,* edited by M. Lewis (Baltimore, MD, Williams & Wilkins, 1991), and a chapter by J. F. Leckman, J. T. Walkup, M. A. Riddle, K. E. Towbin, and D. J. Cohen in the book *Psychopharmacology: The Third Generation of Progress,* edited by H. Y. Meltzer (New York, Raven, 1987). The author wishes to thank Bradley S. Peterson, M.D., and David E. Walker for their comments on an earlier version of this chapter.

act, and a need to perform tics or compulsions until they are felt to be "just right."

Although TS was once thought to be a rare condition, recent epidemiologic studies indicate that between 0.1% and 0.6% of boys are affected with this disorder. The prevalence of TS among girls is substantially lower, perhaps by as much as an order of magnitude (0.01% to 0.06%).

Tourette's syndrome is a familial condition. Twin and family studies have confirmed that vulnerability to TS is genetically determined. These studies have further suggested that in some instances obsessive-compulsive disorder (OCD) may arise from the same underlying genetic diathesis as does TS. Mathematical models of genetic transmission lend support to this conclusion and suggest that the putative gene for TS may be transmitted as an autosomal dominant trait. International efforts to localize the TS gene are currently underway.

Studies of monozygotic twins have indicated that nongenetic factors are critically involved in the expression of TS. A variety of factors have been implicated, including prenatal events and exposures to stress, central nervous system (CNS) stimulants, or psychoactive steroids.

The neurobiological substrates of TS have not been fully determined. There is a substantial body of data that implicates the basal ganglia and related cortical and thalamic structures in the pathobiology of both TS and OCD. These data include findings from neuroimaging studies; case reports describing neurosurgical interventions or injuries involving cortico-striato-thalamocortical circuits; and a large body of neurochemical and neuropharmacological studies of the neurotransmitter and neuromodulatory systems found in these brain regions.

In providing care and treatment, it is important to recall that tic disorders are chronic, if not lifelong, conditions. Continuity of care is desirable and should be considered before embarking on a course of treatment. Standard treatment modalities include education and supportive interventions and treatment with psychopharmacological agents. Typically, patients with chronic motor tics alone do not require drug treatment. For individuals with TS and OCD, it is often desirable to treat the comorbid OCD as a first step, particularly if the OCD symptoms are more severe. Psychoanalytically oriented or cognitive-based psychotherapy can be a useful adjunct in selected cases. Behavioral and dietary treatments have not yet provided consistent positive effects.

The rapidly increasing knowledge base in human genetics and the neurosciences makes it likely that fundamental advances will be made in our understanding of TS during the next decade. The localization and characterization of the vulnerability gene in TS would be a major advance and would lead the way to improved diagnostic procedures, as well as the development of novel, effective treatment approaches.

The relationship between TS and some forms of OCD is heuristically important, as it suggests that OCD may be etiologically heterogeneous. Forms of OCD that are related to TS may be distinct from the remaining types of OCD in terms of natural history, prognosis, and pattern of treatment response. Future research will need to address these possible distinctions and establish whether or not determination of TS relatedness will advance our understanding of the phenomenology, pathophysiology, and treatment of this subgroup of OCD patients.

Phenomenology of Tics and Tourette's Syndrome–Related Obsessions and Compulsions

Definitions

A *tic* is a sudden, repetitive movement, gesture, or utterance that typically mimics some aspect of normal behavior. Usually of brief duration, individual tics rarely last more than a second. They tend to occur in bouts and at times have a dramatic paroxysmal character. Individual tics can occur singly or together in an orchestrated collage. They vary in their intensity or forcefulness. Although many tics can be temporarily suppressed, they are frequently experienced as being involuntary. They may be associated with somatic sensory urges that are relieved with the performance of the tic. Motor tics vary from simple abrupt movements such as eye blinking, head jerks, or shoulder shrugs, to more complex, purposive-appearing behaviors such as facial expressions and gestures of the arms or head. In extreme cases, these movements can be obscene (copropraxia) or self-injurious (e.g., hitting or biting). Phonic or vocal tics can range from simple throat-clearing sounds to more complex vocalizations and speech. In severe cases, coprolalia (obscene speech) is present.

It can be extremely difficult to distinguish between complex motor tics and compulsions. Similarly, the conscious awareness of somatosensory urges may be difficult to differentiate from obsessive thoughts. One a priori approach to distinguishing *tic*-related obsessions and compulsions from *classical* obsessions and compulsions is presented in Table 6–1. In this approach to organizing clinical observations, the premonitory somatosensory urges are viewed as a tic-related obsessive symptom, while touching, tapping, and picking are designated as tic-related compulsive behaviors. "Evening-up" phenomena (i.e., those in which bodily sensations must be bilaterally and symmetrically equivalent) and other perceptually guided compulsions (i.e., behaviors that must be repeated until they look, feel, or sound "just right") also are included in this category.

Nosology of Tic Disorders

Tic disorders are frequently chronic conditions that can impair self-esteem, family life, social acceptance, and school or job perfor-

---

Table 6–1.   Obsessive-compulsive symptoms in Tourette's syndrome

Obsessive thoughts

Tic related: Recurrent, unwanted sensory urges or thoughts associated with tics; thoughts that the sequence of tics needs to be "just right."

Independent of tics: Intrusive, repugnant thoughts or images about death, sexual matters, religious beliefs, unrelated to the tics, that lead to efforts to "resist" them and that are associated with marked distress or interference.

Compulsive behaviors

Tic related: Stereotyped complex "tics" of tapping, picking, sniffling, touching (objects, self, others), kissing, copropraxia, hitting, biting (self), "evening up."

Independent of tics: Counting, ordering rituals, washing, dressing, and/or checking rituals, that classically are performed according to certain rules and that are not an end in themselves but are intended to prevent mental distress or some imagined catastrophe.

---

mance. Individuals with tic disorders may manifest a broad array of behavioral difficulties including disinhibited speech and conduct, impulsivity, distractibility, motoric hyperactivity, and obsessive-compulsive symptoms. Some of these associated "non-tic" symptoms may be a major source of impairment.

Although tic symptoms have been reported since antiquity, systematic study dates only from the 19th century with the reports of Itard (1825) and Gilles de la Tourette (1885). Gilles de la Tourette, in his classic study of 1885, described nine cases of tic disorder characterized by motor "incoordinations" or tics, as well as "inarticulate shouts accompanied by articulated words with echolalia and coprolalia" (Gilles de la Tourette 1885). This report also hinted both at the association between tic disorders and obsessive-compulsive symptoms and at the hereditary nature of the syndrome.

The current classification of tic disorders in DSM-III-R (American Psychiatric Association 1987) includes Tourette's disorder or syndrome, chronic motor or vocal tic disorder, transient tic disorder, and tic disorder not otherwise specified. The criteria for the first three of these conditions are presented in Table 6–2. These criteria focus on the phenomenology and natural history of the disorder and are readily applied in clinical settings. They also serve as the basis for the diagnostic descriptions contained in the World Health Organization's Tenth Revision of the International Classification of Diseases (World Health Organization 1988). Several conditions, including intoxication syndromes and known CNS disease such as Huntington's chorea and postviral encephalitis, preclude a diagnosis of TS using DSM-III-R criteria. The presence of OCD, however, does not exclude a TS diagnosis.

Natural History of Tourette's Syndrome

The most severe tic disorder is best known by the eponym "Gilles de la Tourette's syndrome." Typically the disorder begins in early childhood with transient bouts of simple motor tics such as eye blinking or head jerks. These tics initially may come and go, but they eventually become persistent and can have adverse effects on the child and his or her family. The repertoire of motor tics can be vast, incorporating virtually any voluntary movement by any portion of the body. Although some authors have drawn attention to a "rostral-caudal" progression of motor tics (head, neck, shoulders, arms, torso), this course is not predictable. As the syndrome develops, complex motor tics may appear. Often they have a "camouflaged" appearance (e.g., brushing hair away from the face with an arm) and

Table 6–2.   Tic disorders: DSM-III-R diagnostic criteria

Tourette's syndrome [disorder] (307.23)

1. Both multiple motor and one or more vocal tics have been present at some time during the illness, although not necessarily concurrently.
2. The tics occur many times a day (usually in bouts), nearly every day or intermittently throughout a period of more than 1 year.
3. The anatomic location, number, frequency, complexity, and severity of the tics change over time.
4. Onset before age 21.
5. Occurrence not exclusively during psychoactive substance intoxication or known central nervous system disease, such as Huntington's chorea and postviral encephalitis.

Chronic motor or vocal tic disorder (307.22)

1. Either motor or vocal tics, but not both, have been present at some time during the illness.
2. The tics occur many times a day, nearly every day, or intermittently throughout a period of more than 1 year.
3. Onset before age 21.
4. Occurrence not exclusively during psychoactive substance intoxication or known central nervous system disease, such as Huntington's chorea and postviral encephalitis.

Transient tic disorder (307.21)

1. Single or multiple motor and/or vocal tics.
2. The tics occur many times a day, nearly every day for at least 2 weeks, but for no longer than 12 consecutive months.
3. No history of Tourette's [syndrome] or chronic motor or vocal tic disorder.
4. Onset before age 21.
5. Occurrence not exclusively during psychoactive substance intoxication or known central nervous system disease, such as Huntington's chorea and postviral encephalitis.

Tic disorder not otherwise specified (307.20)

Tics that do not meet the criteria for a specific tic disorder. An example is a tic disorder with onset in adulthood.

Source. Reprinted with permission from American Psychiatric Association *Diagnostic and Statistical Manual of Mental Disorders,* 3rd Edition, Revised. Washington, DC, American Psychiatric Association, 1987, American Psychiatric Association.

can only be distinguished as tics by their repetitive character. Occasionally complex motor tics can be self-injurious and further complicate management (e.g., punching one side of the face or biting a wrist).

On average, phonic tics begin 1 to 2 years after the onset of motor symptoms and are usually simple in character (e.g., throat clearing, grunting, squeaks). More complex vocal symptoms such as echolalia, palilalia, and coprolalia occur in a minority of cases. Other complex phonic symptoms include dramatic and abrupt changes in vocal rhythm, rate, and volume.

Both motor and phonic tics tend to occur in bouts. Their frequency ranges from nonstop bursts that are virtually uncountable, to rare events that occur only a few times a week. Single tics may occur in isolation, or there may be well-orchestrated combinations of motor and phonic tics that involve multiple muscle groups.

The forcefulness of motor tics and the volume of phonic tics can also vary tremendously, from behaviors that are not noticeable (e.g., a slight shrug or a hushed guttural noise), to strenuous displays that are frightening and exhausting (e.g., arm thrusts or loud barking).

Consistent with available epidemiologic data, tic disorders tend to improve in late adolescence and early adulthood. In many instances, the phonic symptoms become increasingly rare or may disappear altogether, and the motor tics may be reduced in number and frequency. Complete remission of both motor and phonic symptoms has also been reported (Bruun 1988; Shapiro et al. 1988). In contrast, adulthood is also the period when the most severe and debilitating forms of tic disorder can be seen.

In addition to the tic behaviors, associated behavioral and emotional problems frequently complicate TS. These difficulties range from impulsive, "disinhibited," and immature behavior to compulsive touching or sniffing.

Comorbidity of Tourette's Syndrome and Obsessive-Compulsive Disorder

Since 1977, a number of investigators have explored the relationship between TS and OCD in clinic samples (Table 6–3). Overall, at least

Table 6–3.   Occurrence of obsessive-compulsive symptoms (OCS) and obsessive-compulsive disorder (OCD) in patients with Tourette's syndrome: clinical studies

Study	N	OCS/OCD
Yaryura-Tobias 1977	55	29
Cohen et al. 1978, 1980	25	56
Nee et al. 1980, 1982	5	68
Montgomery et al. 1982	12	67
Min 1983	24	17
Lees et al. 1984	53	61
Grad et al. 1987	25	28
Frankel et al. 1986	63	52
Comings and Comings 1987	250	35
Shapiro et al. 1988	666	3–63
Bruun 1988	350	16–42
Robertson et al. 1988	90	37
Bornstein et al. 1990	763	8–85
Pauls et al. 1991	86	36

30% to 40% of adult TS subjects have some obsessive-compulsive features. The rates are lower in pediatric samples. However, it is difficult to generalize from these data given the varying assessment techniques and the selection biases at work in clinical samples.

Epidemiology

Tic behaviors are commonplace among children. Community surveys indicate that 1% to 13% of boys and 1% to 11% of girls manifest "frequent . . . tics, twitches, mannerisms or habit spasms" (Zahner et al. 1988). The instability of these estimates is in part due to the wording of items on symptom inventories, the identity of the informant, and the demographic characteristics of the sample studied. Children between the ages of 7 and 11 years appear to have the highest rates. Although boys are more commonly affected with tic behaviors than girls, the male-female ratio in most community surveys is less than 2 to 1. Urban living may be associated with elevated rates (Zahner et al. 1988). Race and socioeconomic status have not been shown to influence the point prevalence of tics.

Much less is known concerning the prevalence of tic disorders.

Although these disorders were once thought to be rare, current estimates from registers of clinically diagnosed subjects suggest that 1% to 2% of the general population may be affected with a tic disorder and 0.01% to 0.6% of the population may have TS, depending on the age and gender of the subjects (Comings et al. 1990; Shapiro et al. 1988). Unfortunately these estimates are likely to be low, as rigorous population-based studies have not been performed. Available data do provide evidence that children are 5 to 12 times more likely to be identified as having a tic disorder than adults, and that males are more commonly affected than females (with male-to-female ratios of 9 to 1 and 3 to 1 for children and adults, respectively) (Burd et al. 1986a, 1986b). Although other demographic characteristics have not been systematically investigated, some authors have suggested that tic disorders may be more common among Caucasian and Asian racial groups.

The Role of Genetic Factors in Tourette's Syndrome and Related Disorders

Twin and family studies provide evidence that genetic factors are involved in the vertical transmission of a vulnerability to TS and related disorders within families (Pauls and Leckman 1988).

Twin Studies

The concordance rate for TS among monozygotic twin pairs is greater than 50%, while the concordance of dizygotic twin pairs approaches 10% (Price et al. 1986; Walkup et al. 1988). If co-twins with chronic motor tic disorder are included, these concordance figures increase to at least 77% for monozygotic and 30% for dizygotic twin pairs. Differences in the concordance of monozygotic and dizygotic twin pairs indicate that genetic factors play an important role in the etiology of TS and related conditions. These figures also suggest that nongenetic factors are critical in determining the nature and severity of the clinical syndrome.

Family Studies

Studies of first-degree family members (i.e., parents, siblings, and offspring) of individuals with TS indicate that these family members are at substantially higher risk for developing TS, chronic motor tic disorder, and OCD than are unrelated individuals (Pauls and Leckman 1986). Overall, the risk to male first-degree family members approximates 50% (18% TS, 31% chronic motor tics, and 7% OCD), while the overall risk to females is less (5% TS, 9% chronic motor tics, and 17% OCD) (Pauls et al. 1991). The basis for these gender-dependent differences in the phenotypic expression is unknown but likely involves a differential response of the developing CNS to gender-specific factors such as steroids produced in gonads and adrenals (see below). The possible contribution of steroids produced in glia, the so-called "neurosteroids," has not been addressed with regard to either TS or OCD.

Application of Genetic Models

The pattern of vertical transmission among family members has led several groups of investigators to test whether or not mathematical models of specific genetic hypotheses could account for these data. The bulk of this work favors models of autosomal dominant transmission (Pauls and Leckman 1988).

Genetic Linkage Studies

The suggestion that the vulnerability to TS and related conditions may be due to a single major autosomal gene has led directly to the identification of large multigenerational families to facilitate genetic linkage studies (Kurlan et al. 1986). Although linkage studies have not yet been successful in determining the chromosomal location of the putative TS gene or genes (Gelernter et al. 1990; Pauls et al. 1990), systematic efforts are underway that should lead to a successful outcome within the next several years.

Other Factors That Influence the Expression of Tourette's Syndrome and Related Disorders

Neuroendocrine Factors

The increased prevalence of TS and other tic disorders among males may be related to the exposure of the developing male CNS to elevated levels of testosterone and/or other gender-specific hormones (Leckman et al. 1984). This hypothesis is based in part on the observation that although TS is more prevalent among males, it does not appear to be transmitted as a sex-linked trait (Pauls and Leckman 1988), for which higher rates among males would be expected. A second line of evidence comes from the observation that the onset and course of tic symptomatology do not appear to be related to activation during puberty of the hypothalamic-pituitary-gonadal axis, as the tic symptoms usually commence well before this period. In addition, anecdotal evidence has implicated androgenic steroids in the exacerbation of TS symptoms among "body builders" who abuse these agents (Leckman and Scahill 1990). It is also intriguing to note that antiandrogens have been reported to have a beneficial effect on OCD symptomatology (Casas et al. 1986). If these findings are confirmed, they point the way to a new understanding of the increased numbers of males affected with TS and open important new approaches to treatment.

Perinatal Factors

The search for nongenetic factors that mediate the expression of a genetic vulnerability to TS and related disorders has also focused on the role of adverse perinatal events. This interest dates from the report of Pasamanick and Kawi (1956), who found that mothers of children with tics were 1.5 times more likely to have experienced a complication during pregnancy than the mothers of children without tics. Other investigators have reported that among monozygotic twins discordant for TS, the index twins with TS uniformly had a lower birth weight than the unaffected co-twins (Leckman et al. 1987a). Severity of maternal life stress during pregnancy and severe nausea and/or vomiting during the first trimester have likewise been implicated as potential risk factors in the development of tic disorders (Leckman et al. 1990). Some of these factors may alter dopamine levels in the developing CNS, and this in turn may have an enduring effect on the number of striatal D_2 receptors in the mature animal (Friedhoff 1986). In contrast, two studies have failed to document any association between adverse perinatal events and manifestations of TS (Shapiro and Shapiro 1988).

Psychological Factors

Tic disorders have long been identified as "stress-sensitive" conditions (Jagger et al. 1982; Shapiro and Shapiro 1988). Typically, symptom exacerbations follow in the wake of stressful life events. As noted by Shapiro, these events need not be adverse in character to produce this effect (Shapiro and Shapiro 1988). Clinical experience suggests that in some unfortunate instances a vicious cycle can be initiated in which tic symptoms are misunderstood by family and teachers, who then actively attempt to discourage the symptoms by punishment and even humiliation. These efforts can lead to a further exacerbation of symptoms and a further increase in stress in the child's interpersonal environment. Unchecked, this vicious cycle can lead to the most severe manifestations of TS and dysthymia as well as maladaptive characterological traits. Although psychoanalytic and dynamic formulations of TS have been largely discredited (Mahler and Rangell 1943), the intimate association of the content and timing of tic behaviors and dynamically important events in the lives of children makes it difficult to overlook the contribution of such events to the intramorbid course of these disorders.

In addition to the intramorbid effects of stress and anxiety that have been well characterized, some authors have suggested that premorbid stress may play an important role as a sensitizing agent in the pathogenesis of TS among vulnerable individuals (Leckman et al. 1984).

Neurobiological Substrates

Neuroanatomical Data

The basal ganglia and related structures in the midbrain and cortex are likely to serve as the neuroanatomical substrate for TS. These speculations are based on the following:

1. An emerging appreciation of the functional interrelationships among these structures and their regulation of sensorimotor activities as well as some aspects of cognitive processing and emotive behaviors
2. Inconclusive neuropathological and neuroimaging studies
3. A large body of neurochemical and neuropharmacological data that implicates some of the neurotransmitter and neuromodulatory systems found in these brain regions.

The basal ganglia have long been recognized as providing a critical way station in the multiple parallel cortico-striato-thalamocortical circuits that concurrently subserve a wide variety of sensorimotor, motor, oculomotor, cognitive, and limbic processes (Goldman-Rakic and Selemon 1990). The emerging picture of each of these circuits being composed of hundreds of minicircuits that channel and subchannel discrete bits of information has been most extensively documented in the motor circuit, in which preparatory and execution-related aspects of motor control may be regulated by the activity of somatotopically arranged subpopulations of neurons (Alexander and Crutcher 1990). TS and etiologically related forms of OCD may be associated with a failure to inhibit subsets of these cortico-striato-thalamocortical minicircuits (Leckman et al. 1991b).

Other aspects of the circuitry of the basal ganglia may provide important clues concerning the anatomic distribution of motor tics and the "choice" of obsessive themes frequently encountered in forms of OCD related to TS. Specifically, the unidirectional input from the amygdala (arising largely from the parvicellular portion of the basal nucleus and the amygdalohippocampal area) to widespread areas of the nucleus accumbens and ventral portions of the caudate and putamen, appears to overlap those areas most affected in TS. Studies in primates and man have also shown that stimulation of the amygdala produces motor and vocal activity reminiscent of the symptoms of TS (Baldwin et al. 1954; MacLean and Delgado 1953).

In addition, reciprocal connections between midbrain sites (periaqueductal gray, substantia nigra, and the ventral tegmental area [VTA]) and structures in the basal ganglia, amygdala, and hypothalamus are likely to play a critical role in the genesis and maintenance of the symptoms of TS (Devinsky 1983). These connections may also contribute to the stress sensitivity of the disorder. The distribution of androgen and estrogen receptors and the existence of sexual dimorphic regions within some of these structures may also account for the more frequent expression of TS in males than in females (Simerly et al. 1990).

Few neuropathological studies have been performed. Balthazar (1956) reported hypoplasia of the corpus striatum (caudate and putamen) with a loss of the interneuronal neuropil. These findings, however, were based on a single case and were not consistent with an earlier report that found no distinctive histological pattern (Dewulf and van Bogaert 1940). Laplane and co-workers (1981, 1989) reported two intriguing case reports of individuals with basal ganglia lesions that were associated with tics, obsessive-compulsive symptoms, and deficits in motivation. More recently, neuroimaging studies have provided limited support for the involvement of the caudate nuclei and the prefrontal cortex in OCD (Baxter et al. 1987) and the involvement of the caudate in TS (Chase et al. 1984, 1986).

Neurochemical Systems and Neuropharmacological Data

The functional status of a number of neurotransmitter and neuromodulator systems has been evaluated in TS. The most compelling evidence has focused attention on nigrostriatal and nigrocortical dopaminergic projections; serotonergic projections from the dorsal raphe to the substantia nigra, globus pallidus and striatum; and peptidergic projections from the striatum to the pallidum and substantia nigra (Leckman et al. 1987b).

Basing his hypothesis largely on parallels between the tics, vocalizations, and obsessive-compulsive behaviors seen in some patients with encephalitis lethargica, Devinsky (1983) has suggested that TS is the result of altered dopaminergic function in the midbrain. The substantia nigra and the VTA are adjacent midbrain sites that contain large numbers of dopaminergic neurons. The dopamine cell bodies in the substantia nigra give rise to the ascending nigrostriatal pathway. The dopaminergic neurons of the VTA send ascending projections to various cortical regions including the anterior cingulate gyrus and other limbic structures. The dopaminergic neurons in the substantia nigra and those of the VTA also give rise to descending pathways projecting to the dorsal pontine tegmentum in the region of the noradrenergic locus coeruleus.

Other data implicating central dopaminergic mechanisms include clinical trials in which haloperidol and other neuroleptics that preferentially block dopaminergic D_2 receptors have been found to be effective in the partial suppression of tics in a majority of TS patients (Shapiro and Shapiro 1988). Friedhoff (1986) has suggested that the relationship between the D_2 and D_1 systems may be of interest in TS, in that blockade of D_2 receptors by relatively selective agents such as haloperidol and pimozide disinhibits the D_1 system.

Tic suppression has also been reported after interventions that limit dopamine synthesis, such as the administration of alpha-methyl-para-tyrosine or tetrabenazine (Leckman et al. 1987b; Shapiro and Shapiro 1988). In contrast, TS-like syndromes have appeared following withdrawal of neuroleptics, and tics are often exacerbated following exposure to agents that increase central dopaminergic activity such as L-dopa and CNS stimulants like cocaine.

These pharmacological data—taken together with reports of lowered baseline and postprobenecid mean CSF levels of homovanillic acid (HVA), a major metabolite of brain dopamine, in TS patients compared with available contrast groups (Butler et al. 1979; Cohen et al. 1978; Leckman and Cohen 1988; Singer et al. 1982)—have led several groups of investigators to suggest that TS is a disorder in which postsynaptic dopaminergic D_2 receptors are hypersensitive. Recent preliminary positron-emission tomography (PET) studies of brain dopamine receptors, however, do not support the view that there are increased numbers of these receptors in the few TS patients who have been studied. Additional imaging studies are needed to address fully the potential abnormalities of receptor number, affinity, and distribution. It is also important to keep in mind that the reported pharmacological effects are partial. Dopaminergic D_2 receptor blocking agents suppress tics, but they do not eliminate them. Overall, these data suggest that the inferred dysfunction in brain dopaminergic D_2 receptors may not be the primary pathophysiological mechanism in tic disorder patients. A full exploration of the possible role of D_1 and D_3 receptors has yet to be undertaken in TS.

Although serotonergic mechanisms have been repeatedly invoked as potentially playing an important role in the pathophysiology of TS, there is very little hard evidence to support this connection. Serotonergic inputs from the dorsal raphe to both the substantia nigra and the striatum have been identified and partially characterized, but there is no direct neuropathological data implicating these areas in TS. Medications that act by increasing or decreasing serotonergic activity do not consistently alter tic symptoms. Studies of cerebrospinal fluid (CSF) 5-hydroxyindoleacetic acid (5-HIAA), the principal central metabolite of serotonin, have reported a range of low and normal levels in TS patients compared with contrast groups (Butler et al. 1979; Cohen et al. 1978; Leckman and Cohen 1988; Singer et al. 1982). Despite this lack of evidence, serotonergic hypotheses continue to be attractive. Circumstantial evidence includes their neuroanatomical projections and their likely involvement in the pathophysiology of OCD.

Endogenous opiates, including dynorphin and met-enkephalin, are highly concentrated in structures of the extrapyramidal system. These neuropeptides are known to interact with central dopaminergic neurons and may play an important role in the control of motor functions (Buck and Yamamura 1982). These systems have also been directly implicated in the pathophysiology of Parkinson's disease, Huntington's disease, and, most recently, TS. The neuropathological study of Haber et al. (1986) reported decreased levels of dynorphin A [1–17] immunoreactivity in striatal fibers projecting to the globus pallidus in the brain of a patient with severe TS. This observation and the separate finding of elevated levels of CSF dynorphin A [1–8] (Leckman et al. 1988), in conjunction with the neuroanatomical distribution of dynorphin and its broad range of motor and behavioral effects, have led to speculation concerning the role of dynorphin in the pathobiology of TS. Additional evidence supporting the role of endogenous opiates comes from the dramatic, but poorly documented effects of opiate antagonists in TS (Sandyk 1985).

Other reports have summarized neurobiological findings in OCD, but they are limited by the lack of direct comparisons between TS and OCD subjects (Hollander et al. 1989) and by the failure of investigators to use family genetic data as a way of identifying OCD subjects whose disorder is etiologically related to TS.

Treatment

Tic disorders are frequently chronic, if not lifelong, conditions. Continuity of care is desirable and should be considered before embarking on a course of treatment. Major treatment modalities include education and supportive interventions, and treatment with neuropsychopharmacological agents. Typically, patients with chronic motor tics alone do not require drug treatment. Psychotherapy can be a useful adjunctive treatment in selected cases. Behavioral and dietary treatments have not yet provided consistent positive effects.

Educational and Supportive Interventions

Although the efficacy of eductional and supportive interventions has not been independently assessed, these interventions seem to have salutary effects by reshaping negative expectations (Cohen et al. 1988). This is particularly true when the tic behaviors have been misconstrued by the family and others as voluntary and intentionally provocative. Families also find descriptions of the natural history comforting, in that the disorders tend not to be relentlessly progressive and usually improve during adulthood. This information often contradicts the impressions gained from the available lay literature on TS, which typically focuses on the most extreme cases. In addition, the presentation of TS as a neuropsychiatric disorder determined by a neurobiological vulnerability and influenced by psychosocial factors can help families fend off the stigmatizing effects of a purely mental disorder. For children, contact with their teachers can be enormously valuable. By educating the educators, clinicians can make significant progress toward securing for the child a positive and supportive environment in the classroom.

Psychopharmacological Treatment

For individuals who are experiencing significant impairment as a result of their tic behaviors, treatment with drugs can provide a source of relief. Although virtually every agent in the *vade mecum psychopharmacologium* has been used in the treatment of TS, only the relatively selective D_2 receptor antagonists haloperidol and pimozide have proven to be effective during the course of rigorous double-blind clinical trials.

Approximately 70% of patients with TS respond favorably to either haloperidol or pimozide (Shapiro et al. 1989), and the mean reduction of symptom severity is also in the range of 70% to 80%. In general, it is useful to start treatment with low doses of medication and to make any necessary increases gradually. Typically treatment is initiated with a low dose (0.25 mg of haloperidol or 1 mg of pimozide) given before sleep. Further increments (0.5 mg of haloperidol or 1 mg of pimozide) may be added at 7- to 14-day intervals if the tic behaviors remain severe. In most instances, 0.5 to 6.0 mg per day of haloperidol or 1.0 to 10.0 mg per day of pimozide administered over a period of 4 to 8 weeks is sufficient to suppress tic symptoms.

Tic symptoms often continue to wax and wane, at a much reduced level, even during periods of neuroleptic treatment. Generally it is not a good idea to "chase" the tic symptoms with adjustments in medication dosage. Such adjustments generally are not beneficial and may expose the subjects to additional unwanted physical effects of the medication, many of which appear to be dose related.

The major limiting factor in the use of neuroleptics is the emergence of side effects, including acute dystonias, akathisia, akinesia, cognitive impairment, and weight gain (Shapiro and Shapiro 1988). A majority of subjects will experience one or more of these effects, and a significant proportion of these subjects will elect to discontinue treatment if the side effects are not controlled. In addition to these effects, pimozide may have an adverse effect on cardiac conduction in some TS subjects, particularly at doses above 10 to 12 mg per day. Tardive dykinesia has also been reported in TS patients with chronic exposure to neuroleptics. Given the short- and long-term hazards of neuroleptics, many clinicians elect to use these medications only in severe cases.

Clonidine, a selective α_2-adrenergic receptor agonist, may be effective for a smaller proportion of TS subjects (Cohen et al. 1979). Clinical trials indicate that subjects can expect on average a 25% to 35% reduction in their symptoms over an 8- to 12-week period (Leckman et al. 1985, 1991a). The usual starting dose is 0.05 mg on arising. Further 0.05-mg increments at 3- to 5-hour intervals are added weekly until a dosage of 5 g per kg is reached or until the total daily dose exceeds 0.25 mg.

Although clonidine is clearly less effective than haloperidol and pimozide, it is considerably safer. The principal side effect associated with its use is sedation, which occurs in nearly all subjects to a mild degree. Only a small proportion (<10%) of subjects experience moderate levels of sedation that require dose reductions. This unwanted physical effect usually abates with continued use. In general, clonidine has not proven to be effective in reducing the obsessive-compulsive symptoms associated with TS and other tic disorders (Leckman et al. 1991a).

Serotonin reuptake inhibitors such as fluoxetine and clomipramine have consistently been reported to be of benefit for the obsessive-compulsive symptoms associated with TS (Riddle et al. 1990). The effect of these drugs can be enhanced by the addition of low-dose neuroleptics such as pimozide (McDougle et al. 1989). To date, however, there has been no convincing demonstration of a beneficial effect of serotonin reuptake inhibitors on tic symptoms (Riddle et al. 1990).

Prognosis

The prognosis for tic disorders is generally good, with most subjects experiencing their worst tic symptoms from ages 10 to 15 years. The course in adulthood is variable, but most subjects report a more or less stable repertoire of tic symptoms that wax and wane over a reduced range of severity.

Poorer prognoses are associated with comorbid developmental and mental disorders, chronic physical illness, unstable and unsupportive family environments, and exposure to psychoactive drugs such as cocaine. Potential complications include the emergence of OCD, character pathology associated with a chronic stigmatizing disorder, and physical injuries secondary to self-abusive motor tics.

Research Directions

As outlined throughout this chapter, a broad array of research opportunities are now being actively pursued. Based largely on advances in related fields of science, genetic and neurobiological studies show particular promise. Progress in these areas will clarify the relationship between TS and OCD and may herald significant advances in early detection and diagnosis as well as advances in treatment for both disorders.

References

Alexander GE, Crutcher MD: Functional architecture of basal ganglia circuits: neural substrates of parallel processing. Trends Neurosci 13:266–271, 1990

American Psychiatric Association: Diagnostic and Statistical Manual of Mental Disorders, 3rd Edition, Revised. Washington, DC, American Psychiatric Association, 1987

Baldwin M, Frost LL, Wood CD: Investigation of primate amygdala: movements of the face and jaws. Neurology 4:586–598, 1954

Balthazar K: Uber das anatomishe substrat der generalisierten tic-krankeit (maladie des tics, Gilles de la Tourette): entwicklungshemmung des corpus striatum. Archiv für Psychiatrie und Nervenkrankheiten 195:531, 1956

Baxter LR, Phelps ME, Mazziota JC, et al: Local cerebral glucose metabolic rates in obsessive-compulsive disorder. Arch Gen Psychiatry 44:211, 1987

Bornstein RA, Stefl ME, Hammond L: A survey of Tourette syndrome patients and their families: the 1987 Ohio Tourette survey. Journal of Neuropsychiatry and Clinical Neurosciences 2:275–281, 1990

Bruun RD: The natural history of Tourette's syndrome, in Tourette's Syndrome and Tic Disorders: Clinical Understanding and Treatment. Edited by Cohen DJ, Bruun RD, Leckman JF. New York, Wiley, 1988, pp 21–40

Buck SH, Yamamura HI: Neuropeptides in normal and pathological basal ganglia. Adv Neurol 35:121–132, 1982

Butler IJ, Koslow SH, Seifert WE Jr, et al: Biogenic amine metabolism in Tourette syndrome. Ann Neurol 6:37–39, 1979

Burd L, Kerbeshian L, Wikenheiser M, et al: Prevalence of Gilles de la Tourette's syndrome in North Dakota adults. Am J Psychiatry 143:787, 1986a

Burd L, Kerbeshian L, Wikenheiser M, et al: A prevalence study of Gilles de la Tourette syndrome in North Dakota school-age children. Journal of the American Academy of Child Psychiatry 25:552, 1986b

Casas M, Alvarez P, Duro C, et al: Antiandrogenic treatment of obsessive-compulsive neurosis. Acta Psychiatr Scand 73:221–222, 1986

Chase TN, Foster NL, Fedio P, et al: Gilles de la Tourette syndrome: studies with the fluorine-18–labeled fluorodeoxyglucose positron emission tomographic method. Ann Neurol 15(suppl):S175, 1984

Chase TN, Geoffrey V, Gillespie M, et al: Structural and functional studies of Gilles de la Tourette syndrome. Rev Neurol (Paris) 142:851–855, 1986

Cohen DJ, Shaywitz BA, Caparulo B, et al: Chronic, multiple tics of Gilles de la Tourette's disease: CSF acid monoamine metabolites after probenecid administration. Arch Gen Psychiatry 35:245, 1978

Cohen DJ, Young JG, Nathanson JA, et al: Clonidine in Tourette's syndrome. Lancet 2:551, 1979

Cohen DJ, Deltor J, Young JG, et al: Clonidine ameliorates Gilles de la Tourette syndrome. Arch Gen Psychiatry 37:1350–1357, 1980

Cohen DJ, Ort SI, Lechman JF, et al: Family functioning and Tourette's syndrome, in Tourette's Syndrome and Tic Disorders: Clinical Understanding and Treatment. Edited by Cohen DJ, Bruun RD, Leckman JF. New York, Wiley, 1988, pp 179–196

Comings DE, Comings BG: A controlled study of Tourette syndrome, IV: obsessions, compulsions, and schizoid behaviors. Am J Hum Genet 41:782–803, 1987

Comings DE, Himes JA, Comings BG: An epidemiologic study of Tourette's syndrome in a single school district. J Clin Psychiatry 51:463–469, 1990

Devinsky O: Neuroanatomy of Gilles de la Tourette's syndrome: possible midbrain involvement. Arch Neurol 40:508, 1983

Dewulf A, van Bogaert L: Etudes anatomo-cliniques de syndromes hyper-cinetiques complexes. Monatsschr Psychiatr Neurol 104:53, 1940

Frankel M, Cummings JL, Robertson MM, et al: Obsessions and compulsions in Gilles de la Tourette's syndrome. Neurology 36:378–382, 1986

Friedhoff AJ: Insights into the pathophysiology and pathogenesis of Gilles de la Tourette syndrome. Rev Neurol (Paris) 142:860, 1986

Gelertner J, Pakstis AJ, Pauls DL, et al: Gilles de la Tourette syndrome is not linked to D2 dopamine receptor. Arch Gen Psychiatry 47:1073–1077, 1990

Gilles de la Tourette G: Étude sur une affection nerveuse caractérisée par de l'incoordination motrice accompagnée d'echolalie et de copralalie. Arch Neurol 9:19–42, 158–200, 1885

Goldman-Rakic PS, Selemon LD: New frontiers in basal ganglia research. Trends Neurosci 13:241–243, 1990

Grad LR, Pelcovitz D, Olson M, et al: Obsessive-compulsive symptomatolgy in children with Tourette's syndrome. Journal of the American Academy of Child Psychiatry 26:69–74, 1984

Haber SN, Kowall NW, Vonsattel JP, et al: Gilles de la Tourette's syndrome: a postmortem neuropathological and immunohistochemical study. J Neurol Sci 75:225–241, 1986

Hollander E, Liebowitz MR, DeCaria CM: Conceptual and methodological issues in the studies of obsessive-compulsive and Tourette's disorders. Psychiatr Dev 4:267–296, 1989

Itard JMG: Memoire sur quelques fonctions involontaires des appareils de la locomotion de la prehension et de la voix. Arch Gen Med 8:385, 1825

Jagger J, Prusoff BA, Cohen DJ, et al: The epidemiology of Tourette's syndrome: a pilot study. Schizophr Bull 8:267–278, 1982

Kurlan R, Behr J, Medved L, et al: Familial Tourette's syndrome: report of a large pedigree and potential for linkage analysis. Neurology 36:772, 1986

Laplane D, Widlocher D, Pillon B, et al: Comportement compulsif d'allure obsessionnelle par necrose circonscrite bilaterale pallido-striatale: en-cephalopathie par piqure de quepe. Rev Neurol (Paris) 137:269–725, 1981

Laplane D, Levasseur M, Pillon B, et al: Obsessive-compulsive and other behavioral changes with bilateral basal ganglia lesions. Brain 112:699–725, 1989

Leckman JF, Cohen DJ: Descriptive and diagnostic classification of tic disorders, in Tourette's Syndrome and Tic Disorders: Clinical Understanding and Treatment. Edited by Cohen DJ, Bruun RD, Leckman JF. New York, Wiley, 1988, pp 3–20

Leckman JF, Scahill L: Possible exacerbation of tics by androgenic steroids. N Engl J Med 322:1674, 1990

Leckman JF, Cohen DJ, Price RA, et al: The pathogenesis of Gilles de la Tourette's syndrome: a review of data and hypothesis, in Movement Disorders. Edited by Shah AB, Shah NS, Donald AG. New York, Plenum, 1984, pp 257–274

Leckman JF, Deltor J, Harcherik D, et al: Short- and long-term treatment of Tourette's disorder with clonidine. Neurology 35:343–351, 1985

Leckman JF, Price RA, Walkup JT, et al: Nongenetic factors in Gilles de la Tourette's syndrome. Arch Gen Psychiatry 44:100, 1987a

Leckman JF, Walkup JT, Riddle MA, et al: Tic disorders, in Psychopharmacology: The Third Generation of Progress. Edited by Meltzer HY. New York, Raven, 1987b, pp 1239–1246

Leckman JF, Riddle MA, Berrettini WH, et al: Elevated CSF dynorphin A [1-8] in Tourette's syndrome. Life Sci 43:2015–2023, 1988

Leckman JF, Dolnansky ES, Hardin MT, et al: Perinatal factors in the expression of Gilles de la Tourette's syndrome: an exploratory study. J Am Acad Child Adolesc Psychiatry 29:220–226, 1990

Leckman JF, Hardin MT, Riddle MA, et al.: Clonidine treatment of Tourette's syndrome. Arch Gen Psychiatry 48:324–328, 1991a

Leckman JF, Knorr AM, Rasmusson AM, et al: Basal ganglia research and Tourette's syndrome. Trends Neurosci 14:94, 1991b

Lees AJ, Robertson M, Timble MR, et al: A clinical study of Gilles de la Tourette syndrome in the United Kingdom. J Neurol Neurosurg Psychiatry 47:1–8, 1984

Mahler MS, Rangell L: A psychosomatic study of maladie des tics (Gilles de la Tourette's disease). Psychiatr Q 17:579, 1943

MacLean PD, Delgado JMR: Electrical and chemical stimulation of frontotemporal portion of the waking animal. Electroencephalogr Clin Neurophysiol 5:91–100, 1953

McDougle CJ, Goodman WK, Price LH, et al: Neuroleptic addition in fluvoxamine-refractory obsessive-compulsive disorder. Yale Psychiatric Quarterly 12:9–10, 1989

Min SK: Gilles de la Tourette syndrome: report on 24 cases. Yonsei Med J 24:76–82, 1983

Montgomery MA, Clayton PC, Friedhoff AJ: Psychiatric illness in Tourette syndrome patients and first-degree relatives, in Gilles de la Tourette Syndrome. Edited by Friedhoff AJ, Chase TN. New York, Raven, 1982, pp 335–340

Nee LE, Caine ED, Polinsky RJ, et al: Gilles de la Tourette syndrome: clinical and family study of 50 cases. Ann Neurol 7:41–49, 1980

Nee LE, Polinsky RJ, Ebert MH: Tourette syndrome: clinical and family studies, in Gilles de la Tourette Syndrome. Edited by Friedhoff AJ, Chase TN. New York, Raven, 1982, pp 291–296

Pasamanick B, Kawi A: A study of the association of prenatal and paranatal factors in the development of tics in children. J Pediatr 48:596–601, 1956

Pauls DL, Leckman JF: The inheritance of Gilles de la Tourette syndrome and associated behaviors: evidence for autosomal dominant transmission. N Engl J Med 315:993, 1986

Pauls DL, Leckman JF: The genetics of Tourette's syndrome, in Tourette's Syndrome and Tic Disorders: Clinical Understanding and Treatment. Edited by Cohen DJ, Bruun RD, Leckman JF. New York, Wiley, 1988, pp 91–

Pauls DL, Pakstis AJ, Kurlan R, et al: Segregation and linkage analysis of Gilles de la Tourette's syndrome and related disorders. J Am Acad Child Adolesc Psychiatry 29:195–203, 1990

Pauls DL, Raymond CL, Stevenson JF, et al: A family study of Gilles de la Tourette syndrome. Am J Hum Genet 48:154–163, 1991

Price AR, Leckman JF, Pauls DL, et al: Tics and central nervous system stimulants in twins and non-twins with Tourette syndrome. Neurology 36:232–237, 1986

Riddle MA, Hardin MT, King RA, et al: Fluoxetine treatment of children and adolescents with Tourette's and obsessive-compulsive disorders. J Am Acad Child Adolesc Psychiatry 29:45–48, 1990

Robertson M, Timble MR, Lees AJ: The psychopathology of Gilles de la Tourette syndrome: a phenomenological analysis. Br J Psychiatry 152:383–390, 1988

Sandyk R: The endogenous opioid system in neurological disorders of the basal ganglia. Life Sci 37:1655–1663, 1985

Shapiro AK, Shapiro ES: Treatment of tic disorders with haloperidol, in Tourette's Syndrome and Tic Disorders: Clinical Understanding and Treatment. Edited by Cohen DJ, Bruun RD, Leckman JF. New York, Wiley, 1988, pp 267–280

Shapiro AK, Shapiro ES, Young JG, et al: Gilles de la Tourette Syndrome, 2nd Edition. New York, Raven, 1988

Shapiro ES, Shapiro AK, Fulop G, et al: Controlled study of haloperidol, pimozide, and placebo for the treatment of Gilles de la Tourette's syndrome. Arch Gen Psychiatry 46:722–730, 1989

Simerly RB, Chang C, Muramatsu M, et al: Distribution of androgen and estrogen receptor mRNA-containing cells in the rat brain. J Comp Neurol 294:76–95, 1990

Singer HS, Tune LE, Butler IJ, et al: Clinical symptomatology, CSF neuro-transmitter metabolites, and serum haloperidol levels in Tourette syn-drome. Adv Neurol 35:177–184, 1982

Walkup JT, Leckman JF, Price AR, et al: The relationship between obses-sive-compulsive disorder and Tourette's syndrome: a twin study. Psy-chopharmacol Bull 24:375–379, 1988

World Health Organization: ICD-10 draft of Chapter V: mental, behavioral, and developmental disorders: clinical descriptions and diagnostic guide-lines. Geneva, World Health Organization, 1988

Yaryura-Tobias JA: L-Tryptophan in obsessive-compulsive disorders. Am J Psychiatry 134:1298–1299, 1977

Zahner GEP, Clubb MM, Leckman JF, et al: The epidemiology of Tourette's syndrome, in Tourette's Syndrome and Tic Disorders: Clinical Under-standing and Treatment. Edited by Cohen DJ, Bruun RD, Leckman JF. New York, Wiley, 1988, pp 79–90

Chapter 7

Sexual Compulsions

Donna T. Anthony, M.D., Ph.D.
Eric Hollander, M.D.

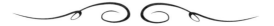

Compulsive sexual behavior includes repetitive sexual acts and intrusive sexual thoughts. The person feels compelled or driven to perform the behavior, which may or may not cause subjective distress. Psychiatric treatment may be sought out of a desire to change the behavior or may be legally mandated, as in the case of some paraphilias. While not ego-dystonic, the behavior may interfere with other aspects of the patient's life. For example, compulsive masturbation may become so time-consuming that it interferes with work or relationships. The threat of AIDS in the last decade has prompted some people to attempt to change their patterns of sexual behavior.

In contrast, sexual obsessions are ego-dystonic, intrusive thoughts about sexual matters that do not usually prompt a sexual behavior. Thus, sexual obsessions can be considered a form of obsessive-compulsive disorder (OCD) itself.

Unlike sexual obsessions, the categorization of the sexual compulsions is more difficult, and there is no consensus among mental health professionals about their treatment. Behavioral treatments yield only partial success with substantial recidivism. The lack of standardized, effective treatments for compulsive sexual behaviors in large part reflects our poor understanding of the etiology of these behaviors. The extent to which these behaviors are truly "compulsive" remains unresolved.

It has been proposed that sexual compulsions exist on a spectrum with OCD-related disorders (Jenike 1989). Because sexual compulsions are initially pleasurable, they do not entirely resemble true compulsions in OCD, which are initially senseless but also temporarily relieve discomfort. Alternatively, compulsive sexual behaviors may be classified with other addictive behaviors. As such, these behaviors might be carried out in response to painful, intolerable affects such as anxiety and depression. While this debate is not new (Coleman 1990; Sprenkle 1987), compelling data have not emerged to resolve it.

Phenomenology

The prevalence of compulsive sexual behaviors is unknown. Our lack of knowledge about the epidemiology of these behaviors in part reflects the fact that only a minority of those who manifest compulsive sexual behavior present for treatment. Far more men than women have been reported to admit to sexual compulsions (Cooper et al. 1990; Weissberg and Levay 1986). It is unclear if there is a real sex bias to these conditions or if men come to the attention of professionals with greater frequency. Alternatively, women may express an underlying condition with different symptomatology. At the moment, any theories about this sex difference in prevalence would be purely speculative.

Three types of behaviors—sexual obsessions, paraphilias, and other sexual compulsions such as promiscuity or compulsive masturbation—are discussed under the broad category of compulsive sexuality and representative examples given below. Hypersexuality that occurs during a manic or hypomanic episode will not be discussed here, as it clearly exists as part of that symptom complex. However, mania and hypomania should be included in the differential diagnosis of hypersexual behaviors, particularly in women.

Although comorbid anxiety, depression, and substance abuse, as well as other disorders of impulse control, have been described, rigorous statistics on comorbidity are not yet available. In one study of persons classifying themselves as "sex addicts," 38% were chemically dependent, and another 38% had eating disorders (Sprenkle 1987). It is likely that one disorder may be primary, with subsequent behaviors or affective syndromes developing in response. Data on family history of sexual compulsions are similarly lacking.

Clinical Examples

Sexual obsessions are persistent, intrusive sexual thoughts or fantasies that are usually distressing to the patient. The patient may be compelled to carry out some ritual to counteract or neutralize the obsession. Increased religious activity sometimes results from the patient's hypermoral reactions to these obsessions.

Case 1: Sexual Obsessions

A 39-year-old man developed a preoccupation with looking at other men's crotches and the fear that he would be discovered (Stein et al., in press). His obsessions led to difficulty making presentations at work and an inability to function in social situations. These intrusive, obsessive thoughts and the resulting compulsion to stare at crotches rendered him chronically anxious and dysphoric and interfered with completion of his work. On fluoxetine, 80 mg a day, the obsessions gradually abated over 14 weeks, with concomitant improvement in his mood.

Paraphilias include unusual or bizarre imagery or repetitive acts generally involving preference for a nonhuman object for sexual arousal, or activities with humans involving suffering or humiliation, or with nonconsenting partners. Patients with paraphilias describe recurrent, repetitive urges to carry out these deviant sexual behaviors. Patients often have more than one paraphilia, and if a dominant paraphilia is treated, another often emerges or intensifies (Abel et al. 1988). Sex offenders with paraphilias, such as rapists and pedophiles, often come to treatment through the legal system and not out of their own desire to break the compulsion.

The paraphilias enumerated in DSM-III-R (American Psychiatric

Association 1987) include exhibitionism (exposing one's genitals to an unsuspecting stranger), fetishism (sexually arousing fantasies and activity involving the use of nonliving objects by themselves), frotteurism (urges and fantasies of touching and rubbing against a nonconsenting person), pedophilia (sexual activity and fantasies involving prepubescent children), sexual masochism (urges and fantasies involving the act of being humiliated, beaten, bound, or otherwise made to suffer), sexual sadism (urges and fantasies involving acts in which the psychological or physical suffering of the victim is sexually exciting), transvestic fetishism (cross-dressing), and voyeurism (urges and fantasies involving the act of observing an unsuspecting person who is naked or involved in sexual activity), among others. The person with a paraphilia may be merely distressed by these urges or may actually act on them.

Case 2: Paraphilia

A 38-year-old man with concomitant OCD reported pleasurable sadomasochistic fantasies with himself as the victim. He masturbated to fantasies of being beaten and mainly had sex with prostitutes who would humiliate him. This patient presented initially only for treatment of his OCD symptoms; he reported improvement in his OCD symptoms on fluoxetine but no change in his sexual behavior (Stein et al., in press).

Additional sexual compulsions include promiscuous sexual behavior and compulsive masturbation. The era of AIDS has prompted many to change a pattern of sexual involvement with multiple partners, although it is often difficult for them to do so voluntarily. Patients with compulsive masturbation often present for treatment because the activity begins to consume many hours a day, interfering with work or a relationship.

Case 3: Other Sexual Compulsions

A 40-year-old man presented with a 10-year history of compulsive masturbation that was associated with humiliating fantasies involving cross-dressing (Stein et al., in press). He described feeling anxious if he could not give in to the compulsion to masturbate, which could occupy him for many hours. He also noted an increased desire to masturbate when facing stressful situations that required him to assert himself. He presented for treatment after he married and felt unable to continue this compulsive behavior in the presence of his wife. He also reported being frequently late to work because of the compulsive behavior, and complained of poor concentration.

Relationship With Obsessive-Compulsive Disorder

Like OCD patients, patients with sexual obsessions also suffer from characteristic intrusive and distressing thoughts or impulses. Their symptoms may be limited to these sexual thoughts, or they may involve a range of other obsessions and compulsions as well.

Paraphilias and sexual compulsions are immediately pleasurable, which is in contrast to the compulsions of OCD, which are usually senseless and disturbing. Sexual compulsions may become distressing when they are time consuming, have legal repercussions, or expose the person to sexually transmitted diseases. The fantasy or activity may embarrass the person or violate his or her ethical standards, but it is initially pleasurable. Both the compulsions of OCD and sexual compulsions are reported to relieve some dysphoric affect, usually anxiety (Qualand 1985; Rapoport 1990). Treatment of the sexual compulsions will be discussed below. In general, behavioral therapies and group therapy have been used with some success (Kilmann et al. 1982; Qualand 1985). Unlike the pharmacotherapy of OCD, for which a number of effective agents now exist, effective pharmacotherapy for sexual compulsions has not yet been established (Hollander 1991).

Etiologies

No simple mechanisms exist to explain sexual compulsions, with current hypotheses ranging from psychodynamic conflicts to addictions. Additionally, given the phenomenological overlap of sexual obsessions and compulsions with OCD symptoms, these disorders may belong to the spectrum of obsessive-compulsive–related disorders (OCRDs) (Coleman 1990; Jenike 1989). Different mechanisms may be operative for sexual obsessions and compulsions.

Sexual compulsions have been described as disorders of impulse control and are not now considered to be related to an abnormally high sex drive (Barth and Kinder 1987; Weissberg and Levay 1986). Many patients become uncomfortable or anxious if they try to prevent these impulses. Likewise, most people describe a release of tension after engaging in the sexual compulsion. Furthermore, the frequency of these behaviors increases during times of life stresses. This response to a dysphoric affect and subsequent relief of tension is also seen in other disorders of impulse control such as compulsive gambling and trichotillomania, two disorders that may also be part of the spectrum of OCRDs (Hollander et al. 1991; see also Chapters 5 and 8, this volume). Patients may have more than one of these compulsive, anxiety-driven behaviors concurrently or sequentially. In addition, patients with Tourette's syndrome who also have obsessive and compulsive features describe a release of tension and the urge to repeat behaviors, which may be sexual, until the patients "feel right," that is, until their anxiety is diminished (Comings and Comings 1987).

The tendency to resort to a typical behavior pattern under stress is also found in substance use disorders and other addictions (Qualand 1985). In patients with sexual compulsions, as in those with addictions, relief of anxiety is fleeting, so the behavior becomes repetitive (Qualand 1985). Levine and Troiden (1988) describe commonly observed features of loneliness, low self-esteem, and anxiety in patients suffering from addictions or disorders of impulse control. Schaffer and Zimmerman (1990) report withdrawal symptoms of anxiety, insomnia, and depression in individuals who attempt to stop the compulsive activity, while also noting that sexual compulsions are found along with other addictions in the same individual.

McConaghy (1983) argues that behavior-completion mechanisms are responsible for sexual compulsions and other compulsive behaviors. Konopacki and Oei (1988) provide a similar behavioral model in which compulsive sexuality is seen as a function of interrupted or frustrated approach behavior. These two models propose a mechanism to explain the repetitive nature of the sexual compulsion but fail to target the underlying event that initiates the behavior.

Some common developmental correlations have been described, such as childhood abuse and neglect leading to feelings of shame coupled with a background of restrictive attitudes about sex (Coleman 1987; Sprenkle 1987). Women who have been sexually abused as children have a high frequency of compulsive sexual behaviors and sadomasochistic fantasies (Craine et al. 1988). Similarly, Young (1990) reports that relapse in sexual compulsions and other addictions can be traced to the uncovering of incest memories. The addiction model hypothesizes that because anxiety and depression are common in patients with sexual compulsions, the sexual behavior provides temporary relief from these painful affects that possibly arise from the above developmental issues.

Thus, sexual compulsions share features of OCD and addictions. In all cases the behavior temporarily relieves some dysphoric affect and provides a decrease of tension. The compulsions of OCD, however, are generally distressing, and the patient is often unable to resist. The sexual compulsions, on the other hand, are immediately pleasurable but may ultimately have negative consequences. In this way, the sexual compulsions resemble other addictions in that the activities are temporarily gratifying. In contrast, sexual obsessions are almost always disturbing, consistent with their classification as symptoms of OCD.

Finally, neurobiological approaches may be used to investigate etiologies. A serotonergic hypothesis of OCD is based upon the selective efficacy of serotonin reuptake blockers (DeVeaugh-Geiss et al. 1989; Liebowitz et al. 1989), as well as cerebrospinal fluid (CSF) studies of serotonin metabolites (Thorén et al. 1990) and biological challenge studies with serotonin agonists (Hollander et al. 1988, 1991; Zohar et al. 1987). Antiandrogen agents have been used with some success in the treatment of both male and female paraphilias (Cooper et al. 1990) and in childhood-onset OCD patients (Leonard 1989). Rarely, compulsive masturbation occurs as an ictal or interictal phenomenon (Jacome and Risko 1983).

Treatment and Implications for Future Research

Comprehensive studies regarding treatment for sexual obsessions and compulsions are not yet available. Various behavioral therapies yield partial success but often result in relapse (Kilmann et al. 1982). Periodic booster sessions are often required for the long-term behavioral treatment of paraphilias. McConaghy et al. (1985) found that use of the behavioral technique of imaginal desensitization diminished compulsive sexuality. They also found decreased anxiety levels in 20 men with paraphilias and other compulsive sexual behaviors who underwent this treatment. Aversion therapies have been utilized for compulsions but do not prove superior to imaginal desensitization (McConaghy et al. 1985). Following their theory of interrupted approach behavior, Konopacki and Oei (1988) reported two cases of paraphilias in which the behavior diminished after initially permitting access to a similar sexual outlet.

Qualand (1985) utilized group therapy for gay and bisexual men who wished to decrease their sexual encounters with multiple partners. He hypothesized that group therapy would be effective because it is beneficial for other addictions, such as substance abuse and overeating. Qualand also found that his participants increasingly became involved in a primary relationship and had lower numbers of partners per month. He postulated that group therapy reduces isolation and anxiety and promotes intimacy among group members.

Twelve-step programs modeled upon Alcoholics Anonymous also exist for "sex addicts" (Coleman 1990). Sprenkle (1987) has described a case in which couples therapy was effective treatment for a man with multiple paraphilias.

There have been no comprehensive studies of individual psychodynamic psychotherapies for the sexual compulsions.

Reports of pharmacological treatments of sexual compulsions are limited. Coleman (1990) reported on a study demonstrating success with fluoxetine in patients admitted to a sexual dependency unit. Perilstein et al. (1991) described three cases of paraphilias in men, two of whom also reported associated compulsive masturbation. Both the paraphilias and the sexual compulsions responded to fluoxetine. In one case, the patient had associated anxiety and depression before treatment with fluoxetine. In two cases, the patients experienced retarded ejaculation and overall diminished sexual desire during fluoxetine treatment but chose to continue the medication because of the substantial reduction in the paraphilias and compulsions. Cesnik and Coleman (1989) published a case report of a paraphilia associated with dysthymia and obsessional thinking that responded to lithium therapy.

In one intriguing case report in the literature, buspirone was used to effectively treat transvestic fetishism associated with chronic anxiety, while alprazolam alleviated only the anxiety. This patient's cross-dressing behavior, which returned while the patient was off buspirone, was associated with decreased frequency of intercourse with his wife (Fedoroff 1988). Buspirone is a serotonin (5-hydroxy-tryptamine) $5-HT_{1A}$ agonist that decreases presynaptic serotonin neurotransmission (Peroutka 1985) and thus differs from other anxiolytics. Fishbain (1989) argues that the patient had an inconclusive trial of alprazolam, and he cites examples of other compulsions or addictions that respond to anxiolytics. Further examination of the effects of buspirone on sexual behavior is warranted.

We conducted a retrospective chart review of 15 patients with sexual obsessions and compulsions (Stein et al., in press). Some of these patients had comorbid OCD, depression, anxiety, or substance abuse diagnoses. Most patients presented to an OCD clinic for treatment, and, in many cases, the sexual compulsions were not the primary complaint. We analyzed the patients' responses to anti-OCD medications such as clomipramine, fluoxetine, and fluvoxamine. Some trends became apparent, although a larger prospective study is needed for replication. Improvement was found when a small sample of patients whose predominant sexual complaint was hyper-moral sexual obsessions were treated with anti-OCD medications. However, in patients with sexual compulsions, only a minority responded to anti-OCD medications. Medication response was often seen only in parallel with alleviation of OCD or depression. Several paraphilias did not respond to anti-OCD medications. At times, trials of these medications were limited by their sexual side effects (Pies 1990).

Conclusions

Compulsive behavior remains difficult to categorize and treat. While sexual obsessions, a subtype of OCD, may respond to serotonergic medications, isolated sexual compulsions have no single definitive treatment. Sexual compulsions such as promiscuity, compulsive masturbation, and paraphilias manifest some features of OCD but in other ways are more like addictions. These compulsions are similar to the compulsions in OCD in that they are driven behaviors that decrease tension. Also, some OCD patients, particularly those with low CSF 5-hydroxyindoleacetic acid (5-HIAA) levels, have strong aggressive and sexual impulses and urges (Leckman et al. 1990). However, sexual compulsions are initially pleasurable and thus resemble other addictive behaviors. The lack of response to serotonin reuptake blockers in our small sample suggests a pharmacological dissection between OCD and sexually impulsive disorders, although other case reports cited above argue against this conclusion. Efficacious treatment of the sexual compulsions may in fact be multidimensional, because widely disparate therapies have been used with some success. Precise characterization of the sexual compulsions should help in the development of definitive treatments.

References

Abel GG, Becker JV, Cunningham-Rathner J, et al: Multiple paraphilic diagnoses among sex offenders. Bull Am Acad Psychiatry Law 16:153–168, 1988

American Psychiatric Association: Diagnostic and Statistical Manual of Mental Disorders, 3rd Edition, Revised. Washington, DC, American Psychiatric Association, 1987

Barth RJ, Kinder BN: The mislabeling of sexual impulsivity. J Sex Marital Ther 13:15–23, 1987

Cesnik JA, Coleman E: Use of lithium carbonate in the treatment of autoerotic asphyxia. Am J Psychother 43:277–286, 1989

Coleman E: Sexual compulsivity: definition, etiology, and treatment considerations, in Chemical Dependency and Intimacy Dysfunction. Edited by Coleman E. New York, Haworth Press, 1987, pp 189–204

Coleman E: The obsessive-compulsive model for describing compulsive sexual behavior. American Journal of Preventive Psychiatry and Neurology 2:9–14, 1990

Comings DE, Comings BG: A controlled study of Tourette syndrome, IV: obsessions, compulsions, and schizoid behaviors. Am J Hum Genet 41:782–803, 1987

Cooper AJ, Swaminath S, Baxter D, et al: A female sex offender with multiple paraphilias: a psychologic, physiologic (laboratory sexual arousal) and endocrine case study. Can J Psychiatry 35:334–337, 1990

Craine LS, Henson CE, Colliver JA, et al: Prevalence of a history of sexual abuse among female psychiatric patients in a state hospital system. Hosp Community Psychiatry 39:300–304, 1988

DeVeaugh-Geiss J, Landau P, Katz R: Treatment of obsessive compulsive disorder with clomipramine. Psychiatric Annals 19:97–101, 1989

Fedoroff JP: Buspirone hydrochloride in the treatment of transvestic fetishism. J Clin Psychiatry 49:408–409, 1988

Fishbain DA: Buspirone and transvestic fetishism (letter). J Clin Psychiatry 50:436–437, 1989

Hollander E: Serotonergic drugs and the treatment of disorders related to obsessive-compulsive disorder, in Current Treatments of Obsessive-Compulsive Disorder. Edited by Pato MT, Zohar J. Washington, DC, American Psychiatric Press, 1991, pp 173–191

Hollander E, Fay M, Cohen B, et al: Serotonergic and noradrenergic sensitivity in obsessive-compulsive disorder: behavioral findings. Am J Psychiatry 145:1015–1017, 1988

Hollander E, DeCaria C, Gully R, et al: Effects of chronic fluoxetine treatment on behavioral and neuroendocrine responses to meta-chloro-phenylpiperazine in obsessive-compulsive disorder. Psychiatry Res 36:1–17, 1991

Jacome DE, Risko MS: Absence status manifested by compulsive masturbation. Arch Neurol 40:523–524, 1983

Jenike MA: Obsessive-compulsive and related disorders—a hidden epidemic. N Engl J Med 321:539–541, 1989

Kilmann PR, Sabalis RF, Gearing ML, et al: The treatment of sexual paraphilias: a review of the outcome research. Journal of Sex Research 18:193–252, 1982

Konopacki WP, Oei TP: Interruption in the maintenance of compulsive sexual disorder: two case studies. Arch Sex Behav 17:411–419, 1988

Leckman JF, Goodman WK, Riddle MA, et al: Low CSF 5-HIAA and obsessions of violence: report of two cases (letter). Psychiatry Res 33:95–99, 1990

Leonard HL: Drug treatment of obsessive-compulsive disorder, in Obsessive-Compulsive Disorder in Children and Adolescents. Edited by Rapoport JL. Washington, DC, American Psychiatric Press, 1989, pp 217–236

Levine MP, Troiden RR: The myth of sexual compulsivity. Journal of Sex Research 25:347–363, 1988

Liebowitz MR, Hollander E, Schneier F, et al: Fluoxetine treatment of obsessive-compulsive disorder: an open clinical trial. J Clin Psychopharmacol 9:423–427, 1989

McConaghy N: Agoraphobia, compulsive behaviours and behaviour completion mechanisms. Aust N Z J Psychiatry 17:170–179, 1983

McConaghy N, Armstrong MS, Blaszczynski A: Expectancy, covert sensitization and imaginal desensitization in compulsive sexuality. Acta Psychiatr Scand 72:176–187, 1985

Perilstein RD, Lipper S, Friedman LJ: Three cases of paraphilias responsive to fluoxetine treatment. J Clin Psychiatry 52:169–170, 1991

Peroutka SJ: Selective interaction of novel anxiolytics with 5-hydroxytryptamine$_{1A}$ receptors. Biol Psychiatry 20:971–979, 1985

Pies R: Psychotropic use can result in sexual dysfunction. Psychiatric Times, March, 1990, pp 28–29

Qualand MC: Compulsive sexual behavior: definition of a problem and an approach to treatment. J Sex Marital Ther 11:121–132, 1985

Rapoport JL: The waking nightmare: an overview of obsessive compulsive disorder. J Clin Psychiatry 51 (no 11, suppl):25–28, 1990

Schaffer SD, Zimmerman ML: The sexual addict: a challenge for the primary care provider. Nurse Pract 15:25–33, 1990

Sprenkle DH: Treating a sex addict through marital sex therapy. Family Relations 36:11–14, 1987

Stein DJ, Hollander E, Anthony DT, et al: Serotonergic medications for sexual obsessions, sexual addictions and paraphilias. J Clin Psychiatry (in press)

Thorén P, Åsberg M, Bertilsson L, et al: Clomipramine treatment of obsessive-compulsive disorder, II: biochemical aspects. Arch Gen Psychiatry 37:1289–1294, 1980

Weissberg JH, Levay AN: Compulsive sexual behavior. Medical Aspects of Human Sexuality 20:129–132, 1986

Young EB: The role of incest issues in relapse. J Psychoactive Drugs 22:249–258, 1990

Zohar J, Mueller EA, Insel TR, et al: Serotonergic responsivity in obsessive-compulsive disorder; comparison of patients and healthy controls. Arch Gen Psychiatry 44:946–951, 1987

Chapter 8

Pathological Gambling

Concetta M. DeCaria, M.S.
Eric Hollander, M.D.

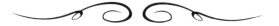

Pathological gambling has only recently been recognized as a distinct entity by the psychiatric community. Increased opportunities for legal and illegal gambling exist, and increasingly younger populations are participating in these activities. For certain individuals, gambling and factors associated with gambling become a dominant part of their lives. These factors often contribute to the deterioration of family and social relationships and to the loss of work, home, and finances. This may lead gamblers to seek illegal resources to temporarily remedy their desperate situation, or may result in personal injury and entanglements with the legal system.

Little is currently known about pathological gambling, and it is frequently overlooked or difficult to identify in a clinical setting. Problems may present as depression or substance abuse. Issues related to gambling, which may have important implications for treatment, are often denied or hidden by the gambler.

In this chapter we present 1) an overview of pathological gambling, 2) its relationship to other disorders, and 3) alternative methods of identification and treatment.

Definition

Defining *pathological gambling* has been a difficult task because it has been characterized as a disorder of impulse control, as a compulsive disorder, and as an addiction. Pathological gambling is classified in DSM-III-R (American Psychiatric Association 1987) as an "Impulse Control Disorder Not Elsewhere Classified." According to DSM-III-R, essential features of pathological gambling are "a chronic and progressive failure to resist impulses to gamble, and gambling behavior that compromises, disrupts, or damages personal, family, or vocational pursuits. The gambling preoccupation, urge, and activity increase during periods of stress. Problems that arise as a result of the gambling lead to an intensification of the gambling behavior" (American Psychiatric Association 1987, p. 324). However, the specificity of the DSM-III-R diagnostic criteria has been challenged.

Rosenthal (1989b) believed that combined diagnostic criteria from DSM-III (American Psychiatric Association 1980) and DSM-III-R would more accurately represent this population. Questionnaires containing diagnostic information from both DSM-III and DSM-III-R were given to 120 people diagnosed with pathological gambling and to a control group of 155 social gamblers. Pathological gamblers differed from control subjects on this questionnaire, and the following diagnostic criteria were proposed for DSM-IV (inclusion of at least three of the following items):

a. Increased preoccupation with gambling as the gambling progresses
b. Development of tolerance and need to increase the amount to sustain level of excitement
c. Withdrawal symptoms, such as irritability, when the gambling behavior decreases
d. Use of gambling as an escape mechanism
e. "Chasing" or returning to gambling after losing in an effort to recover lost money
f. Lying or being deceitful in an attempt to protect oneself from significant others' knowledge of the gambling behavior
g. Involvement in illegal activity to maintain gambling activity

h. Loss or deterioration of personal and social relationships and/or vocational endeavors

i. Dependence on others for continuous "bail outs" from financial dilemmas

In DSM-III, pathological gambling was described as a "Disorder of Impulse Control Not Elsewhere Classified." The essential features of this class of disorders included a) a failure to resist the behavior in question (i.e., gambling), b) an "increasing sense of tension" prior to the behavior, and c) an "experience of either pleasure, gratification, or release" at the time of the behavior. Using DSM-III diagnostic criteria, associations of pathological gambling with compulsive and addictive behavior can be seen. Both compulsive and addictive behavior may be associated with increased levels of tension prior to engaging in the addictive or compulsive activity, and a sense of relief following the activity. For example, for the cocaine user, increased tension and anxiety may accompany the urge to ingest the substance, and, at least for a short period of time, relief occurs. The crash-and-craving cycle of cocaine abuse has its own psychological and physiological mediating factors (Hollander et al. 1990b). However, this may schematically resemble the perceived tension behavior release of the tension/sense-of-pleasure cycle that also occurs during the earlier stages of pathological gambling. Rather than the chemical agent itself, for pathological gamblers, the perceived arousal as a result of the behavior may be regarded as the addictive agent (Anderson and Brown 1984). Pathological gambling also shares aspects associated with addictions, including tolerance (Dickerson 1984), dependence (Moran 1970), and withdrawal (Wray and Dickerson 1981). Unlike addictions, pathological gambling is a disorder that is not readily apparent and is an illness that can be hidden for many years.

In this last regard, pathological gambling is very much like obsessive-compulsive disorder (OCD). In pathological gambling, as in OCD, the tension and anxiety that arise from the obsessive thoughts are relieved by performance of the compulsive behavior. However, in OCD, the ritualistic behavior is described as ego-dystonic. In the case of pathological gambling, as in cocaine addiction, there is a strong sense of pleasure that accompanies the completion of the behavior and the release of tension, at least in the initial stages of the disorder. For this reason, the use of "compulsive gambling" has been questioned and a preference for the label "pathological gambling" has been made (Moran 1970).

Tourette's syndrome is also characterized by a perceived tension felt prior to the expression of motor or vocal tics and a sense of relief of the tension following the release of the behavior (see Chapter 6). Like OCD, this behavior does not seem to be associated with a pleasure state. Trichotillomania, also a disorder of impulse control, is likewise characterized by a recurrent failure to resist impulses to pull out one's own hair. An associated sense of relief of tension following the behavior is sometimes accompanied by a sense of pleasure (see Chapter 5).

Theoretical perspectives, behavioral factors, and biological mechanisms may link these disorders together along a spectrum of impulsivity and compulsivity.

Epidemiology

Two nationwide surveys have provided estimates of the prevalence of pathological gambling in the general population. An American national survey (Commission on the Review of the National Policy Toward Gambling 1976) suggested that 68% of the general population participates in some form of gambling and that 0.77% of American adults are considered probable pathological gamblers. In England, estimates of pathological gambling range from 0.2% (Dickerson 1974) to 1% (Royal Commission on Gambling 1976–1978). State surveys provide prevalence estimates of 1.4% to 3.4% for probable pathological gambling (Commission on the Review 1976; Culleton 1985; Sommers 1988; Volberg and Steadman 1988, 1989).

Although there are methodological problems comparing prevalence estimates based on surveys using various diagnostic criteria and diagnostic instruments, and further studies are needed, certain consistencies remain. However, prevalence estimates in the general population may differ from those estimates derived from people seeking treatment. Volberg and Steadman (1988) compared 6-month estimates of pathological gamblers in treatment programs at three sites in the state of New York with estimates from a New York State general population survey. In the statewide epidemiologic survey, there were more women (36% vs. 7%), younger patients (38% vs. 18%), and more black and Hispanic individuals (43% vs. 9%), with lower income and less education, than in treatment programs. Differences may be a function of changes in the population at risk, or they may represent a biased profile from a select group of patients in treatment. Many individuals who might benefit from treatment may not have the awareness or resources to do so, and existing treatment facilities are minimal.

Estimates of pathological gambling among high school students range from 1.7% to 3.6% (Ladouceur and Mireault 1988), to a high of 5.7% (Lesieur and Klein 1987). Eighty-six percent of those students had gambled within the previous year, and 32% gambled at least once a week. Among college students, estimates of pathological gambling range from 4% to 6% (Frank 1988; Lesieur and Blume 1987). Most pathological gamblers began their gambling career during adolescence (Custer 1982; Livingston 1974), suggesting that early identification and intervention are needed. Among prisoners in New Jersey and Michigan, 30% could be considered probable pathological gamblers (Lesieur and Klein 1985).

Clinical Profile/Comorbidity

Early characteristics associated with pathological gambling include the following (Taber 1980):

♦ Preoccupation with gambling
♦ Excessive gambling
♦ Spontaneous and solitary gambling
♦ Special "gambling money"
♦ Fantasies of success
♦ Increased risk tolerance
♦ Egotism
♦ Denial that gambling behavior could be a problem

Other common characteristics include (Bergler 1943)

◆ Maintaining gambling as a primary interest to the exclusion of other interests
◆ Continuation of gambling behavior while winning and a failure to stop while losing
◆ Apparent lack of understanding of the consequences from the self-defeating behavior and an associated perceived sense of optimism and belief that winning is inevitable
◆ Subjective experience of excitement and tension that is involved in gambling behavior just prior to the outcome of a wager

A general psychiatric profile has been outlined by Blaszczynski and McConaghy (1988). When administered the SCL-90, a 90-item self-report that has been strongly correlated with the Minnesota Multiphasic Personality Inventory (MMPI) (Derogatis 1977), pathological gamblers had low scores on factors pertaining to obsessive-compulsiveness, sensitivity, anxiety, and phobias, when compared with healthy control subjects. Scores on somatization, hostility, paranoid ideation, and psychoticism were comparable to those of the healthy control subjects. Depression scale scores were elevated for pathological gamblers. Scores on the depression and psychopathy subscales of the MMPI were elevated (Bolen et al. 1975; Graham and Lavenfeld 1985; Moravec and Munley 1983). Pathological gamblers also had elevated depression scores on the Beck Depression Inventory (Lyons 1984).

These clinical profiles have been substantiated by several investigations. In inpatient samples of pathological gamblers, 76% met criteria for a major depressive disorder, and in 14% depression preceded pathological gambling (McCormick et al. 1984). Thirty-eight percent had hypomania; 8% had mania; 2% had schizoaffective disorder, depressed type; and 8% had no disorder. In outpatient samples, 72% became depressed upon stopping, 28% met the criteria for a major depressive disorder, 24% had bipolar disorder, 28% had anxiety disorders, and 52% had alcohol abuse/dependency (Linden et al. 1986). However, in a study that did not use structured interviews, very few patients diagnosed for pathological gambling had mood disorders (Lesieur and Blume 1990).

Hopelessness and suicidality have also been associated with pathological gambling (Linden et al. 1986). Estimates of suicide attempts in this population range from 17% to 24% (Ciarrocchi and Richardson 1989; Custer and Custer 1978; Lesieur 1988; Livingston 1974). Younger patients tended to meet criteria for major depressive disorder and to have suicidal tendencies (McCormick et al. 1984).

Pathological gambling has also been strongly associated with substance abuse and dependency. Nine percent of inpatient substance abusers were diagnosed as pathological gamblers (Lesieur and Blume 1987), and 17% of alcohol abusers had gambling problems (Haberman 1969). Conversely, 47% of pathological gamblers in an inpatient treatment program for gambling also had a diagnosis of alcohol/drug abuse (McCormick et al. 1984). Among Gamblers Anonymous members, 8% abused alcohol and 2% had a drug addiction (Custer and Custer 1978). Fifty-two percent of Gamblers Anonymous members had comorbid drug/alcohol abuse (Linden et al. 1986).

Few studies have specifically looked at female pathological gamblers. One-third of pathological gamblers are female (Lesieur 1988). In one sample of female compulsive gamblers, 24% were compulsive overspenders, 20% compulsive overeaters, and 12% sexually compulsive. In addition, 28% had alcoholic fathers and 5% had alcoholic mothers, while 14% had fathers who were pathological gamblers and 4% had mothers who were pathological gamblers.

Pathological gambling has also been associated with dissociative states. Jacobs (1989) described similar dissociative states among pathological gamblers, compulsive overeaters, and alcohol abusers while each group was involved in the addictive behavior—findings that differed significantly from those among healthy control subjects. Jacobs (1984) compared pathological gamblers to social gamblers on measures of dissociative-like states, including a) the feeling of being in a trance during or shortly after gambling, b) the feeling of being "outside oneself" and watching oneself during or shortly after gambling, c) the feeling of having another identity during or shortly after gambling, and d) the experiencing of a "memory blackout" for a period during or shortly after gambling. Of the pathological gamblers in the sample, 60% to 76% experienced some type of dissociative state compared with 24% of social gamblers. Increased life stressors increased the frequency of perceived dissociative states. Jacobs (1982) suggested that dissociative states may be associated with increased sympathetic arousal and that gambling may precipitate physiological and neurochemical changes that contribute to these states.

However, dissociative states associated with pathological gambling, compulsive overeating, and alcohol abuse may be qualitatively different from dissociative states associated with depersonalization disorder. Depersonalization disorder consists of persistent or recurrent episodes of dissociation of sufficient severity to cause marked distress. Dissociative states in pathological gamblers may be transient, occurring only during or shortly after gambling. This may, however, only reflect the timing during which the questions were asked. Dissociative states may be associated with relief of tension or dysphoria. Hollander et al. (1990a) have noted a relationship between depersonalization disorder and OCD (see Chapter 2). Coexistent OCD with depersonalization disorder was associated with good response to serotonin reuptake blocker treatment. Further investigation may offer insights into some of the neurochemical factors that mediate dissociative states associated with pathological gambling.

There is great variability in the clinical profile of the pathological gambler. Some individuals may gamble in response to other symptoms. For others, clinical syndromes may result from continuous gambling activity. Greater understanding of the heterogeneity of this diagnosis may lead to the development of better methods of identification and more effective treatments.

Clinical Course

A three-phase model of the clinical course of pathogical gambling has been proposed (Custer and Milt 1985) and includes 1) a winning phase; 2) a losing phase, and 3) a desperation phase. This model has been revised to include a social dimension as well as gender specificity (Lesieur and Blume 1990, in press; Rosenthal 1986a, 1989a).

In the *winning phase* (Phase 1) male gamblers associate gambling skills with initial successes and may have a "big win." Preoccupation with gambling and the size of the bets increase. Female gamblers may view gambling as an escape from life's problems or as an anesthetic, as in a dissociative state (Jacobs 1988; Lesieur 1988), accompanied by excitement. Some female gamblers gamble to seek action and often experience a "big win."

The *losing phase* (Phase 2) occurs when the gambler begins to gamble in an effort to recover losses produced by irrational gambling. The gambler often gambles alone. The frequency and the amount of gambling increase. Lying and deceit begin to take place. Disruption of personal, familial, social, occupational, and financial interests occurs. The gambler may then seek out family members for a "bail out."

The *desperation phase* (Phase 3) is characterized by a drastic change in behavior. Involvement in illegal activities such as forgery, fraud, theft, or embezzlement occurs in an effort to sustain gambling activity. The gambler becomes restless and irritable, even abusive to family members at times. Almost all other activities and interests are ignored. At this point, eating and sleeping habits deteriorate. Often suicidal thoughts occur, and sometimes suicide attempts are made.

A fourth phase, the *giving up phase,* has been described (Rosenthal 1989a). During this phase, the pathological gambler comes to the realization that gambling no longer serves the purpose of winning back losses. The gambler realizes that the debts are so outrageous that they will never be settled. This is also the time during which the gamblers become involved in the legal system and are sometimes incarcerated. The gambler is out of control and seems to need external sources to assist in the cessation of the gambling activity.

Life stressors that may precipitate heavy gambling for a person considered a social gambler, or hasten the intensity with which a pathological gambler gambles, include substance use or abuse, death or divorce, birth of a child, threat of or actual physical trauma, and success or failure in an occupational setting (Bolen and Boyd 1968; Boyd and Bolen 1970). These factors, however, may be contributing factors at only one particular point in time; but for the pathological gambler, the course is chronic, with increasingly devastating consequences as the disorder progresses. Several theories have been proposed, as discussed below, in an attempt to explain why pathological gamblers continue to gamble, despite the consequences.

Theoretical Perspectives

Psychoanalytic, cognitive, behavioral, and physiological theories of pathological gambling have emerged. Each perspective has its own merits and its own limitations. An interactive approach toward understanding the underlying mechanisms of this disorder may be most useful.

Although a psychoanalytic model of pathological gambling has been criticized for its shortcomings, including small and selected samples and untestable assertions (Allcock 1986), these early ideas have provided a conceptual basis for current thinking. Gambling has been associated with 1) masochism, anal fixation, and compulsive personality traits (Von Hattingberg 1914); 2) the desire for excitement, losing as a mechanism for punishing oneself for the guilt experienced for having negative feelings about the father, and an expression of addictive behavior based on a compulsion to masturbate (Freud 1928[1927]/1961); 3) rebellion against parental authority (Bergler 1943); 4) a mechanism to alleviate depression (Greenson 1947; Israeli 1935); and 5) a sense of omnipotence (Bergler 1957; Greenson 1947; Rosenthal 1986a, 1986b).

Others have investigated the cognitive dimensions of pathological gambling. In one sample, more than 80% of gamblers expressed irrational thoughts and inadequate perceptions about certain aspects of the gambling activity, regardless of the type of gambling activity (Gaboury and Ladouceur 1989). Gamblers often attribute losses to chance or irrational external factors and attribute wins to special skills or other attributes of the gambler (Gilovitch 1983).

Gambling behavior can also be viewed based on a model of operant conditioning and a behavior-completion model. Most pathological gamblers have a significant win early in their career. It is the variable reinforcement schedule that drives the pathological gambler to continue to gamble (Bolen and Boyd 1968). The exposure and availability increase the probability of the development of pathological gambling. The arousal associated with the gambling activity becomes the reinforcing agent, for after the initial stages of gambling winning money becomes a secondary factor.

The *optimum level of stimulation model* (Zuckerman 1979a) suggests that every individual has an optimum level of arousal at which he or she feels well and functions most effectively. The arousal may include autonomic as well as cortical arousal that is regulated by environmental stimulation. Increased or decreased levels of stimulation may be sought in an effort to maintain homeostasis. The pathological gambler's search for a continuous increase in arousal may occur intermittently and over time (Zuckerman 1969). Withdrawal symptoms may be experienced and associated with the cessation of gambling and decreased levels of arousal. This model offers an explanation for the continued gambling behavior after intermittent reinforcement patterns have been extinguished.

Gambling sessions often continue until all of one's money is gone. Jacobs (1982, 1984) suggests that there are several reasons why gambling is so resistant to extinction despite increased negative consequences. There is a significant positive reinforcement factor early in the gambler's career as a result of the pleasurable aspect for a person who feels particularly low and deprived. Extremely strong associations have occurred by the extensive repetitions of behavior, both in reality and in fantasy. The most critical factor refers to the nearly phobic-like avoidance of the return to and maintenance of the dysregulated resting state. The contrast is dramatic and seems only to further reinforce the behavior.

The *behavior-completion mechanism hypothesis* (McConaghy 1983) emphasizes that a neural network is associated with the activation of a particular stimulus that has been previously associated with a particular behavior. Once the stimulus begins to activate the system, the behavior pattern must be completed. If there is an interruption of this process, one is left with a stressor interpreted as a noxious event. This hypothesis may apply to pathological gambling. Pathological gambling is not usually stopped in the middle of a string of losses. If so, the gambler may experience increased tension that can then be relieved by the completion of the behavior. This model can be applied to other related disorders such as OCD and Tourette's syndrome.

In OCD, the interruption or prevention of a compulsive urge or action can create tension and anxiety that is perceived as aversive. The completion of certain rituals provides someone with OCD a temporary release of certain anxieties associated with the obsessional thinking or with the compulsive act itself. Another related disorder, Tourette's syndrome, may also be viewed from the behavior-completion model. Often, persons with Tourette's syndrome, or even those individuals with simple tics, can temporarily and willfully withhold the urge to exhibit motor or vocal tics. This often occurs when one is in a public setting. However, it is apparent that volitional control is transient and that dyscontrol is associated with the development of increased tension and an increased urge to express the tics, especially in a familiar setting.

Considerable controversy exists in the literature regarding the volitional aspects of each of these behaviors. In pathological gambling, the volitional aspect of gambling behavior becomes a paramount issue when a gambler becomes involved with the legal system for committing an illegal act, such as embezzling money or writing bad checks, because of the need to have more money with which to gamble. This issue of volition is currently being battled in the state and federal courts. No clear determination has been made, and it is a difficult issue to address. Implications are widespread and can change or sustain the way in which many other illegal acts are viewed. In OCD the compulsive urges and rituals likewise seem to be volitional, as is evidenced in the successful behavioral treatment of OCD. However, training that deals with dissociating the anxiety *and* the obsessions, which often initially provokes the compulsive urges and rituals, must be addressed in order for the treatment to be successful. Behavior therapy is not always successful in reducing the compulsive urges or ritualistic behavior, and the person with OCD is often left with what could be described as a display of the behavior-completion mechanism. In Tourette's syndrome the volitional quality of the expression of a tic, especially of a complex tic, is argued. What is sometimes considered a complex tic is also sometimes regarded as a compulsion. These distinctions have implications for treatment because tics generally respond to dopamine blockers, and compulsions to serotonin reuptake blockers.

A theory of addiction is also associated with pathological gambling. Dependency develops over time to alleviate stress. A dysregulated physiological resting state (either aroused or depressed) may predispose people to addictions (Jacobs 1986). A second factor may involve a childhood feeling of inadequacy. Onset is viewed as being precipitated by a chance occurrence of the addictive stimulus in a person who has these predisposing factors. The behavior is then maintained over time. Compulsive behavior may be a guard against anticipation of anxiety or pain (Jacobs 1982, 1984).

Personality Profile/Dimensional Variables

Identifying personality traits of pathological gamblers helps to discern morbid risk, pathophysiology, and treatment outcome. Unfortunately, the literature is inconsistent. Heterogeneity, sample size and selection, varied assessment scales, and paucity of available research may account for this inconsistency. Personality traits may vary according to the associated types of gambling a gambler chooses. For example, Blaszczynski et al. (1986b) reported that plasma ß-endorphin levels did not significantly differ at baseline between a group of pathological gamblers and normal control subjects. Yet, subgroups of the pathological gamblers differed on this measure. Horse-race gamblers had lower ß-endorphin levels compared with gamblers who used slot machines. One may speculate that different types of gambling attract different personality types. These differences may be associated with levels of arousal produced by gambling, corresponding to one's internal arousal regulatory mechanisms.

Personality profiles of pathological gamblers may incorporate the following dimensions:

1. Impulsivity versus compulsivity
2. Sensation seeking versus risk aversion
3. Extroversion versus introversion
4. Depressed versus nondepressed state

Generally, impulsivity dominates the impulsive-compulsive spectrum in pathological gambling. In pathological gamblers, elevated scores reflecting impulsivity were seen on the Barratt Impulsiveness Scale (Swyhart 1976), the California Personality Inventory (McCormick et al. 1987), and the Millon Multiaxial Inventory (Millon 1983). However, one study did not find between-group differences on the Barratt Impulsiveness Scale (Allcock and Grace 1988), and another found elevated compulsivity scores on the Millon Multiaxial Inventory (Millon 1983).

Although pathological gamblers have been described as sensation seeking (Custer 1982), some studies do not support this view. Significantly lower scores were found on the Thrill and Adventure subscale, the Experience subscale, and the total score on the Zuckerman Sensation-Seeking Scale (Form V), suggesting a decreased tendency toward physical and dangerous activities and a decreased preference for changes in life-style and cognitive stimulation (Allcock and Grace 1988; Blaszczynski et al. 1986a).

Pathological gambling may also be viewed along dimensions of depression, boredom proneness, and extroversion. Elevated scores were found on the Beck Depression Inventory and on the Boredom Proneness Scale (Allcock and Grace 1988; Blaszczynski et al. 1990). However, scores on the Boredom Susceptibility subscale of the Zuckerman Sensation-Seeking Scale were not elevated. Scores on the Eysenck Personality Inventory extroversion scale have been inconsistent (Koller 1972; Moran 1970; Seager 1970), which may reflect variability in sample selection and in the types of gambling preferred. Adding dimensional variables to biological correlates may further define the profile of the pathological gambler.

Biological Correlates

Attempts have been made to identify possible biological correlates of various personality characteristics believed to be associated with pathological gambling. Specifically, biological correlates of impulsivity, inattention, extroversion, and sensation-seeking behavior have been investigated, and interesting findings have emerged.

Electrophysiological, neuropsychological, and biochemical measures may reflect impulsivity and inattention. Electroencephalographic abnormalities, primarily in the frontal and temporal areas, have been found (Stegman et al. 1991) and may be associated with impulse dyscontrol and inattention. Neuropsychological tests have implicated impairment in conceptual thinking and interference control, which may reflect inattention and impulsivity. These electroencephalographic and neuropsychological results are similar to those found in children with attention-deficit disorder (Carlton and Goldstein 1987; Goldstein et al. 1985) and suggest a possible relationship between attention-deficit disorder and pathological gambling.

Biological measures may also reflect impulsivity. Low cerebrospinal fluid (CSF) levels of the serotonin metabolite 5-hydroxyindoleacetic acid (5-HIAA) may be associated with poor impulse control (Linnoila et al. 1983; Roy et al. 1986a, 1986b, 1987a, 1987b; Virkkunen et al. 1987). Measures of brain serotonin cannot, however, be easily gauged from CSF 5-HIAA levels. Further assessment of the role of central serotonin sensitivity in impulsivity may involve biological challenges with serotonergic agents.

The relationship between pathological gambling and impulsivity was examined by determining CSF 5-HIAA levels (Roy et al. 1988). It was hypothesized that the CSF 5-HIAA levels would be low, but this hypothesis was not confirmed. Sampling bias may have occurred, because DSM-III criteria required exclusion of pathological gamblers who also had a diagnosis of antisocial personality disorder. Antisocial personality disorder is associated with poor impulse control, and exclusion of this group may have contributed to these findings.

This study demonstrated that pathological gamblers had significantly higher CSF levels of 3-methoxy-4-hydroxyphenylglycol (MHPG), a metabolite of norepinephrine, and significantly greater urinary outputs of norepinephrine than did control subjects. Urinary MHPG and sensation-seeking scores have been positively correlated in a sample of healthy control subjects (Buchsbaum et al. 1981). Sensation-seeking traits may underlie risk-taking behavior (Zuckerman 1979b, 1984; Zuckerman et al. 1983), and these characteristics may be associated with increased tonic activity of the central noradrenergic system of the pathological gambler (Roy et al. 1988). Caution should be used when interpreting these results in view of the earlier discussion regarding the validity of the relationship between pathological gambling and sensation-seeking characteristics.

The relationship between extroversion, arousal, and pathological gambling has also been investigated (Roy et al. 1989b). Despite the fact that the studies described earlier have not consistently shown elevated scores on the extroversion scale of the Eysenck Personality Questionnaire (EPQ), significant correlations were found between extroversion scores and both CSF and plasma levels of MHPG, urinary outputs of vanillylmandelic acid, and urinary outputs of norepinephrine and its major metabolites (Roy et al. 1989a). There were no significant correlations between the neuroticism and psychoticism scores on the EPQ and plasma levels of norepinephrine or MHPG, or CSF levels of MHPG. This is a curious finding because these are the factors that were associated with pathological gambling more consistently than were the extroversion scores on the EPQ.

Roy has proposed an interesting model based on his findings of psychobiological correlates of pathological gambling. Roy suggests that extroversion, reflected by Eysenck's model (Eysenck 1967), is affiliated with the variability that exists within each individual's arousal system. Because the noradrenergic system has been associated with arousal (Fuxe et al. 1970; Usdin and Snyder 1973), and because pathological gambling has been associated with increased arousal (Anderson and Brown 1984; Boyd 1976; Brown 1986, 1987; Commission on the Review 1976; Dickerson et al. 1987), the noradrenergic system may be implicated in the pathophysiology of pathological gambling. Roy poses an important question related to neurobiological substrates of pathological gambling and asks whether or not they represent a transient state associated with the disorder or an enduring trait associated with pathological gambling. Subsequent biological studies need to be done to further clarify this idea.

Treatment

Few treatment options and treatment facilities for the pathological gambler exist at this time. Self-help groups are the resources that are most available to the gambler. There are few specialized inpatient rehabilitation facilities or outpatient clinics for this population. Effective treatment for pathological gambling is still in the process of being developed (see Chapter 11).

Treatment options thus far have focused on psychoanalysis, behavior and cognitive therapy, self-help group support, and pharmacotherapy. However, most of what is reported about the efficacy of a particular treatment modality has been based on case studies. Very few well-controlled treatment outcome studies are available. Investigations of long-term follow-up are limited.

The earliest reports come from the psychoanalytic literature. Most of the studies that report success in treating pathological gambling are based on single-case studies (Eissler 1950; Harris 1964; Linder 1950; Simmel 1920). Although reports of successful treatment have also been described using larger samples (Bergler 1957), methodological flaws, including biased sampling, lack of outcome criteria, and inadequate assessment of follow-up, contribute to questionable results and clinical significance (Allcock 1986).

Behavioral methods have been used most often as a form of treatment. Gambling is viewed as a learned behavior that can be treated with counter-conditioning. Aversive therapy has been most commonly used (Victor and Krug 1967). The goal of behavior therapy is the total abstinence of gambling behavior. Gamblers Anonymous supports this notion. However, studies of successful controlled gambling have been reported (Dickerson and Weeks 1979; Rankin 1982). Most behavioral treatment studies are not controlled, comparative studies. Instead, they are small-sample or single-case studies primarily using in vivo aversive therapy techniques. In outcome studies at 1-year follow-up, 2 of 3 patients (Barker and Miller 1968), 5 of 14 patients (Seager 1970), 8 of 12 patients (Koller 1972), and a single case (Goorney 1968) reported abstinence.

Combinations of various behavioral interventions have also been used with some apparent success and include self-administered shock, behavior substitution, time-out from family, self-recording of the gambling activity (Cotler 1971), direct punishment, mildly aversive stimuli (rubber-band snapping), and covert desensitization (Greenberg and Rankin 1982). Imaginal desensitization was more effective in decreasing gambling urges and levels of anxiety than was aversive therapy (McConaghy et al. 1983). Aversive therapy techniques are seldom used today as a form of treatment of pathological gambling.

Behavioral techniques may decrease or stop specific gambling behaviors just as they sometimes stop specific compulsions or tics. However, the therapy may not generalize to other behavioral responses that may exist or develop as a substitute for the diminished compulsive or gambling behavior. For example, many patients with OCD describe the emergence of a new compulsion following the reduction or absence of a particular old compulsion. For the gambler, if the specific gambling activity has been extinguished, other behaviors may emerge, such as substance abuse. Often, the underlying internal drive that seems so resistant to treatment continues to act as a force that makes disorders like these difficult to treat behaviorally.

Cognitive therapy has been used with some success in the treatment of pathological gambling. These techniques focus on the arousal associated with gambling. In a preliminary study, the use of cognitive restructuring showed a decrease in the frequency of gambling and associated irrational verbalizations (Ladouceur 1990). Further investigation is needed.

Self-help groups have been available to nearly all gamblers seeking this type of support. Gambling is viewed as a progressive illness that can be stopped. Retrospective studies show a drop-out rate of up to 70% within the first year (Stewart and Brown 1988). Eight percent of the members reported total abstinence at a 1-year follow-up and 7% at a 2-year follow-up (Brown 1985). Success rates are minimal, and the reliability of outcome measures is questionable. It is obvious that self-help groups do not address the treatment needs of a large proportion of those who are seeking help for pathological gambling.

Inpatient treatment and rehabilitation programs have emerged since the early 1970s (Glen 1976; Taber 1981). These programs are modeled after inpatient treatment programs for the rehabilitation of substance abusers. Outcome studies in a sample of pathological gamblers have shown that approximately 55% of patients reported abstinence at 1-year follow-up (Russo et al. 1984; Taber et al. 1987).

Because these are not controlled studies, however, it is difficult to say whether or not spontaneous recovery occurred and contributed to the reported success rate from these groups. In one study, those patients who reported abstinence also reported decreased depression, increased financial stability, increased interpersonal relationships, and an increased likelihood to participate in Gamblers Anonymous or other treatment programs (Russo et al. 1984). However, in another study on pathological gambling, 18% of the patients who were abstinent reported a significant increase in family life and work setting, but were still significantly depressed. This suggests that for some, depression may be associated with the consequence and outcome of gambling, whereas for others gambling may be a consequence or an attempt to deal with depression.

There is a paucity of research on the effectiveness of pharmacotherapy in the treatment of pathological gambling. Of the few studies done, lithium carbonate reportedly demonstrated mild success for those gamblers who also suffered from an affective disorder (Moskowitz 1980). This is an area of research that shows much promise given the high rates of comorbid disorders as well as what appears to be some of the underpinnings relating to the pathophysiology of this disorder. Given the possible overlap of pathological gambling and OCD, controlled trials of serotonin reuptake blockers are needed.

It is apparent that continued efforts need to be made to investigate the effectiveness of specific treatment methods. Well-defined controlled studies with sample sizes large enough to give both clinical and statistical significance are awaiting.

Conclusions

Pathological gambling is a relatively common disorder. Little is known about its etiology. The course is progressive and chronic. Methods for identifying risk factors have not yet been clearly defined. Theoretical perspectives have presented paths for further investigation. Few controlled studies have provided information regarding effective methods of intervention. Complications of pathological gambling include suicide attempts, other self-destructive behavior, legal difficulty, and emotional, social, personal, and financial chaos within the family. Effective treatment requires the gambler to gain an awareness and a sense of control over his or her own impulses and resultant behavior. The identification and treatment of related disorders may help the conceptual development of more effective treatment strategies. Pathological gambling shares features with disorders of impulse control, addictive disorders, and OCD. Further work is needed to clarify where on the impulsivity-compulsivity spectrum pathological gambling lies.

References

Allcock CC: Review: pathological gambling. Aust N Z J Psychiatry 20:259–265, 1986

Allcock CC, Grace DM: Pathological gamblers are neither impulsive nor sensation-seekers. Aust N Z J Psychiatry 22:307–311, 1988

American Psychiatric Association: Diagnostic and Statistical Manual of Mental Disorders, 3rd Edition. Washington, DC, American Psychiatric Association, 1980

American Psychiatric Association: Diagnostic and Statistical Manual of Mental Disorders, 3rd Edition, Revised. Washington, DC, American Psychiatric Association, 1987

Anderson G, Brown R: Real and laboratory gambling, sensation-seeking and arousal. Br J Psychol 75:401–411, 1984

Barker JC, Miller M: Aversion therapy for compulsive gambling. J Nerv Ment Dis 146:285–302, 1968

Bergler E: The gambler: a misunderstood neurotic. Journal of Criminal Psychopathology 4:379–393, 1943

Bergler E: The Psychology of Gambling. New York, International Universities Press, 1957

Blaszczynski AP, McConaghy N: SCL-90 assessed psychopathology in pathological gamblers. Psychol Rep 62:547–552, 1988

Blaszczynski AP, Wilson AC, McConaghy N: Sensation-seeking and pathological gambling. Br J Addict 81:113–117, 1986a

Blaszczynski AP, Winter SW, McConaghy N: Plasma endorphin levels in pathological gamblers. Journal of Gambling Behavior 2:3–14, 1986b

Blaszczynski AP, McConaghy N, Frankova A: Boredom proneness in pathological gambling. Psychol Rep 67:35–42, 1990

Bolen DW, Boyd WH: Gambling and the gambler: a review and preliminary findings. Arch Gen Psychiatry 18:617–630, 1968

Bolen DW, Caldwell AB, Boyd H: Personality traits of pathological gamblers. Paper presented at the Second National Conference on Gambling, South Lake Tahoe, NV, June 1975

Boyd WH: Excitement: the gambler's drug, in Gambling and Society. Edited by Eadington W. Springfield, IL, Charles C Thomas, 1976

Boyd WH, Bolen DW: The compulsive gambler and spouse in group psychotherapy. Int J Group Psychother 20:77–90, 1970

Brown RIF: The effectiveness of Gamblers Anonymous, in The Gambling Studies: Proceedings of the Sixth National Conference on Gambling and Risk Taking. Edited by Eadington WR. Reno, NV, Bureau of Business and Economic Research, University of Nevada, 1985

Brown R: Arousal and sensation-seeking components in the general explanation of gambling and gambling addictions. Int J Addict 21:1001–1016, 1986

Brown R: Classical and operant paradigms in the management of gambling addictions. Behavioural Psychotherapy 15:111–122, 1987

Buchsbaum M, Goodwin F, Muscettola G: Urinary MHPG, stress response, personality factors, and somatosensory evoked potentials in normal subjects and patients with affective disorders. Neuropsychobiology 7:212–224, 1981

Carlton OL, Goldstein L: Physiological determinants of pathological gambling, in Handbook of Pathological Gambling. Edited by Galski T. Springfield, IL, Charles C Thomas, 1987, pp 111–122

Ciarrocchi J, Richardson R: Profile of compulsive gamblers in treatment: update and comparisons. Journal of Gambling Behavior 5:53–65, 1989

Commission on the Review of the National Policy Toward Gambling: Gambling in America. Washington, DC, U.S. Government Printing Office, 1976

Cotler SB: The use of different behavioral techniques in treating a case of compulsive gambling. Behavior Therapy 2:579–584, 1971

Culleton RP: A Survey of Pathological Gamblers in the State of Ohio. Philadelphia, PA, Transition Planning Associates, 1985

Custer RL: An overview of compulsive gambling, in Addictive Disorders Update: Alcoholism, Drug Abuse, and Gambling. Edited by Carone PA, Yoles SF, Kieffer SN, et al. New York, Human Sciences Press, 1982, pp 107–124

Custer RL, Custer LF: Characteristics of the recovering compulsive gambler: a survey of 150 members of Gamblers Anonymous. Paper presented at the Fourth National Conference on Gambling, Reno, NV, December 1978

Custer RL, Milt H: When Luck Runs Out. New York, Facts on File, 1985

Derogatis LR: SCL-90 Administration, Scoring and Procedures Manual: The Revised Version. Baltimore, MD, Johns Hopkins University School of Medicine, 1977

Dickerson MG: The effect of betting shop experience on gambling behavior. Unpublished doctoral dissertation, University of Birmingham, 1974

Dickerson MG: Compulsive Gamblers. London, Longman, 1984

Dickerson MG, Weeks D: Controlled gambling as a therapeutic technique for compulsive gamblers. J Behav Ther Exp Psychiatry 10:139–141, 1979

Dickerson M, Hinchy J, Falve J: Chasing, arousal and sensation seeking in off-course gamblers. Br J Addict 82:673–680, 1987

Eissler KR: Ego-psychological implications of psychoanalytic treatment of delinquents. Psychoanal Study Child 5:97–121, 1950

Eysenck HJ: The Biological Basis of Personality. Springfield, IL, Charles C Thomas, 1967, pp 34–74

Frank M: Casino gambling and college students: three sequential years of data. Paper presented at the Third National Conference on Gambling Behavior, New York, May 1988

Freud S: Dostoevsky and parricide (1928[1927]), in The Standard Edition of the Complete Psychological Works of Sigmund Freud, Vol 21. Translated and edited by Strachey J. London, Hogarth, 1961, pp 173–196

Fuxe K, Hokfelt T, Ungerstedt U: Morphological and functional aspects of central monoamine neurons, in International Review of Neurobiology, Vol 13. Edited by Pfeiffer CC, Smythies J. New York, NY, Academic, 1970, pp 93–126

Gaboury A, Ladouceur R: Erroneous perceptions and gambling. Journal of Social Behavior and Personality 4:411–420, 1989

Gilovitch T: Biased evaluation and persistence in gambling. J Pers Soc Psychol 44:1110–1126, 1983

Glen AM: The treatment of compulsive gamblers at the Cleveland VA Hospital, Brecksville Division. Paper presented at the annual convention of the American Psychological Association, Washington, DC, September 1976

Goldstein L, Manowitz P, Nora R, et al: Differential EEG activation and pathological gambling. Biol Psychiatry 20:1232–1234, 1985

Goorney AB: Treatment of a compulsive horse race gambler by aversion therapy. Br J Psychiatry 114:329—333, 1968

Graham JR, Lavenfeld BH: Personality dimension of the pathological gambler. Journal of Gambling Behavior 2:58–66, 1985

Greenberg D, Rankin H: Compulsive gamblers in treatment. Br J Psychiatry 140:364–366, 1982

Greenson RR: On gambling. American Imago 4:61–77, 1947

Haberman PW: Drinking and other self-indulgences: complements or counter-attractions? Int J Addict 4:157–167, 1969

Harris HI: Gambling addiction in an adolescent male. Psychoanal Q 33:513–525, 1964

Hollander E, Liebowitz MR, DeCaria C, et al: Treatment of depersonalization with serotonin reuptake blockers. J Clin Psychopharmacol 10:200–203, 1990a

Hollander E, Nunes E, DeCaria CM, et al: Dopaminergic sensitivity and cocaine abuse: response to apomorphine. Psychiatry Res 33:161–169, 1990b

Israeli N: Outlook of a depressed patient, interested in planned gambling, before and after his attempt at suicide. Am J Orthopsychiatry 5:57–65, 1935

Jacobs DF: Factors alleged as predisposing to compulsive gambling. Paper presented at the annual convention of the American Psychological Association, Washington, DC, August 1982

Jacobs DF: Study of traits leading to compulsive gambling, in Sharing Recovery Through Gamblers Anonymous. Los Angeles, CA, Gamblers Anonymous, 1984, pp 227–233

Jacobs DF: Factors alleged as predisposing to compulsive gambling. Paper presented at the Annual Convention of the American Psychological Association, Washington, DC, 1982

Jacobs DF: A general theory of addictions: a new theoretical model. Journal of Gambling Behavior 2:15–31, 1986

Jacobs DF: Evidence for a common dissociative-like reaction among addicts. Journal of Gambling Behavior 4:27–37, 1988

Jacobs DF: A general theory of addictions: rationale for and evidence supporting a new approach for understanding and treating addictive behaviors, in Compulsive Gambling: Theory, Research, and Practice. Edited by Shaffer H, Stein SA, Gambino B, et al. Lexington, MA, DC Heath, 1989, pp 35–61

Koller KM: Treatment of poker-machine addicts by aversion therapy. Med J Aust 1:742–745, 1972

Ladouceur R: Cognitive activities among gamblers. Paper presented at the annual convention of the American Association of Behavior Therapy, San Francisco, CA, November 1990

Ladouceur R, Mireault C: Gambling behavior among high school students in the Quebec area. Journal of Gambling Behavior 4:3–12, 1988

Lesieur HR: The female pathological gambler, in The Gambling Studies: Proceedings of the Seventh International Conference on Gambling and Risk Taking. Edited by Eadington WR. Reno, NV, Bureau of Business and Economic Research, University of Nevada, 1988

Lesieur H, Blume SB: The South Oaks Gambling Screen (the SOGS): a new instrument for the identification of pathological gamblers. Am J Psychiatry 144:1184–1188, 1987

Lesieur HR, Blume SB: Characteristics of pathological gamblers identified among patients on a psychiatric admissions service. Hosp Community Psychiatry 41:1009–1012, 1990

Lesieur HR, Blume SB: When lady luck loses: women and compulsive gambling, in Feminist Perspectives on Treating Addictions. Edited by van den Bergh N. New York, Springer, 1991

Lesieur H, Klein R: Prisoners, gambling, and crime. Paper presented at the annual meeting of the Academy of Criminal Justice Sciences, Las Vegas, NV, April 1985

Lesieur HR, Klein R: Pathological gambling among high school students. Addict Behav 12:129–135, 1987

Lesieur HR, Blume SB, Zoppa R: Alcoholism, drug abuse and gambling. Alcoholism (N Y) 10:33–38, 1986

Linden RD, Pope HG Jr, Jones JM: Pathological gambling and major affective disorder: preliminary findings. J Clin Psychiatry 47:201–203, 1986

Linder RM: The psychodynamics of gambling. Annals of the American Academy of Political and Social Sciences 269:93–107, 1950

Linnoila M, Virkkunen M, Scheinin M, et al: Low cerebrospinal fluid 5-hydroxyindoleacetic acid concentration differentiates impulsive from non-impulsive violent behavior. Life Sci 33:2609–2614, 1983

Livingston J: Compulsive Gamblers: Observations on Action and Abstinence. New York, Harper Torchbooks, 1974

Lyons JC: Differences in sensation-seeking and in depression levels between male social gamblers and male compulsive gamblers, in The Gambling Studies: Preceedings of the Sixth National Conference on Gambling and Risk Taking. Edited by Eadington WR. Reno, NV, Bureau of Business and Economic Research, University of Nevada, 1984

McConaghy N: Agoraphobia, compulsive behaviours and behaviour completion mechanisms. Aust N Z J Psychiatry 17:170–179, 1983

McConaghy N, Armstrong MS, Blaszczynski A, et al: Controlled comparison of aversive therapy and imaginal desensitization in compulsive gambling. Br J Psychiatry 142:366–372, 1983

McCormick RA, Russo AM, Ramirez LF, et al: Affective disorders among pathological gamblers seeking treatment. Am J Psychiatry 141:215–218, 1984

McCormick RA, Taber J, Kruedelback N, et al: Personality profiles of hospitalized pathological gamblers: the California Personality Inventory. J Clin Psychol 43:521–527, 1987

Millon T: Millon Clinical Multiaxial Inventory Manual. Minneapolis, MN, National Computer Systems, Interpretive Scoring Systems, 1983

Moran E: Pathological gambling. Br J Hosp Med 4:59–70, 1970

Moravec JD, Munley PH: Psychological test findings on pathological gamblers in treatment. Int J Addict 18:1003–1009, 1983

Moskowitz JA: Lithium and lady luck: use of lithium carbonate in compulsive gambling. N Y State J Med 80:785–788, 1980

Rankin H: Control rather than abstinence as the goal in the treatment of excessive gambling. Behav Res Ther 20:185–187, 1982

Rosenthal RJ: Chance, luck, fate, and destiny: toward a developmental model of pathological gambling. Keynote address of the Second Annual Conference on Gambling Behavior of the National Council on Compulsive Gambling, Philadelphia, PA, November 1986a

Rosenthal R: The pathological gambler's system of self-deception. Journal of Gambling Behavior 2:108–120, 1986b

Rosenthal RJ: Compulsive gambling. Paper presented to the California Society for the Treatment of Alcoholism and Other Drug Dependencies, San Diego, CA, November 1989a

Rosenthal RJ: Pathological gambling and problem gambling: problems in definition and diagnosis, in Compulsive Gambling: Theory, Research, and Practice. Edited by Shaffer H, Stein SA, Gambino B, et al. Lexington, MA, DC Heath, 1989b

Roy A, Virkkunen M, Guthrie S, et al: Indices of serotonin and glucose metabolism in violent offenders, arsonists, and alcoholics, in Psychobiology of Suicidal Behavior. Edited by Mann JJ, Stanley M. Ann N Y Acad Sci 487:202–220, 1986a

Roy A, Virkkunen M, Guthrie S, et al: Monoamines, glucose metabolism, suicidal and aggressive behaviors. Psychopharmacol Bull 22:661–665, 1986b

Roy A, Nutt D, Virkkunen M, et al: Serotonin, suicidal behavior, and impulsivity. Lancet 2:949–950, 1987a

Roy A, Virkkunen M, Linnoila M: Reduced central serotonin turnover in a subgroup of alcoholics. Prog Neuropsychopharmacol Biol Psychiatry 11:173–177, 1987b

Roy A, Adinoff B, Roehrich L, et al: Pathological gambling: a psychobiological study. Arch Gen Psychiatry 45:369–373, 1988

Roy A, Custer R, Lorenz V, et al: Personality factors and pathological gambling. Acta Psychiatr Scand 80:37–39, 1989a

Roy A, De Jong J, Linnoila M: Extraversion in pathological gamblers: correlates with indexes of noradrenergic function. Arch Gen Psychiatry 46:679–681, 1989b

Royal Commission on Gambling, Vol 1. London, Her Majesty's Stationary Office, 1976–1978

Russo AM, Taber JI, McCormick RA, et al: An outcome study of an inpatient treatment program for pathological gamblers. Hosp Community Psychiatry 35:823–827, 1984

Seager CP: Treatment of compulsive gamblers by electrical aversion. Br J Psychiatry 117:545–553, 1970

Simmel E: Psychoanalysis of the gambler. Int J Psychoanal 1:352–353, 1920

Sommers I: Pathological gambling: estimating prevalence and group characteristics. Int J Addict 23:477–490, 1988

Stegman M, Regard M, Landis T, et al: Pathological gambling: neuropsychological and EEG findings. Paper presented at the annual meeting of the International Neuropsychology Society, San Antonio, TX, February 1991

Stewart RM, Brown RIF: An outcome study of Gamblers Anonymous. Br J Psychiatry 152:284–288, 1988

Swyhart PR: The relationship of pathological gambling to money management, impulsiveness and wager preferences. Unpublished doctoral dissertation, California School of Professional Psychology, San Diego, CA, 1976

Taber J: The early detection of pathological gambling. Paper presented at Gamblers Anonymous/Gam-Anon Eastern Regional Conference, Catskill, NY, May 1980

Taber JI: Group psychotherapy with pathological gamblers. Paper presented at the Fifth National Conference on Gambling and Risk Taking, South Lake Tahoe, NV, June 1981

Taber JI, McCormick RA, Russo AM, et al: Follow-up of pathological gamblers after treatment. Am J Psychiatry 144:757–761, 1987

Usdin E, Snyder S (eds): Frontiers in Catecholamine Research. Elmsford, NY, Pergamon, 1973

Victor RG, Krug CM: "Paradoxical intention" in the treatment of compulsive gambling. Am J Psychother 21:808–814, 1967

Virkkunen M, Nuutila A, Goodwin FK, et al: Cerebrospinal fluid monoamine metabolite levels in male arsonists. Arch Gen Psychiatry 44:241–247, 1987

Volberg RA, Steadman HJ: Refining prevalence estimates of pathological gambling. Am J Psychiatry 145:502–505, 1988

Volberg RA, Steadman HJ: Prevalence estimates of pathological gambling in New Jersey and Maryland. Am J Psychiatry 146:1618–1619, 1989

Von Hattingberg H: Analerotik, angstlust und eigensinn. Internationale Zeitschrift für Ärztliche Psychoanalyse 2:244–258, 1914

Wray I, Dickerson MG: Cessation of high frequency gambling and "withdrawal" symptoms. Br J Addict 76:401–405, 1981

Zuckerman M: Theoretical formulations, I, in Sensory Deprivation: Fifteen Years of Research. Edited Zubek JP. New York, Appleton-Century-Crofts, 1969, pp 407–432

Zuckerman M: Sensation-Seeking: Beyond the Optimal Level of Arousal. Hillsdale, NJ, Lawrence Erlbaum, 1979a, pp 12–56

Zuckerman M: Sensation-seeking and risk taking, in Emotions in Personality and Psychopathology. Edited by Izard CE. New York, Plenum, 1979b

Zuckerman M: Sensation-seeking: a comparative approach to a human trait. Behav Brain Sci 7:413–471, 1984

Zuckerman M, Ballenger J, Jimerson D, et al: A correlational test in humans of the biological models of sensation seeking, impulsivity, and anxiety, in Biological Bases of Sensation-Seeking, Impulsivity, and Anxiety. Edited by Zuckerman M. Hillsdale, NJ, Lawrence Erlbaum, 1983, pp 229–248

Chapter 9

Impulsive Personality Disorders and Disorders of Impulse Control

Richard J. Kavoussi, M.D.
Emil F. Coccaro, M.D.

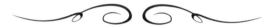

The causes of human impulsivity and aggressivity have eluded behavioral scientists for more than a century. However, syndromes characterized by these behaviors received little attention until the inclusion of specific disorders of impulse control, such as intermittent explosive disorder, pyromania, kleptomania, and pathological gambling, among others, in the DSM-III in 1980 (American Psychiatric Association 1980). Personality disorders with prominent features of impulse dyscontrol (e.g., borderline personality disorder) were similarly neglected until the adoption of operationalized criteria for the diagnosis of these disorders (Spitzer et al. 1979).

Despite the increased attention these disorders have received in the past 10 years, disorders of impulse control remain among the least understood in modern psychiatry. The symptoms of these disorders are a source of frustration to patients with impulse dyscontrol, to those who interact with them, and to the clinicians who treat them. Of increasing interest and optimism, however, is evidence that these disorders may share common psychobiological and treatment-responsive features. Moreover, these features may be shared with features of better-known disorders such as alcoholism, substance abuse, and obsessive-compulsive disorder (OCD). After reviewing current knowledge regarding the phenomenology, etiology, familial transmission, and treatment of the impulsive personality and impulse control disorders, we will present a rationale for their inclusion within a continuum of impulsive-compulsive disorders.

Phenomenology

In DSM-III-R (American Psychiatric Association 1987, p. 321), impulse control disorders (other than the paraphilias and substance abuse) are defined by the following criteria:

1. Failure to resist an impulse to perform some act that is harmful to the individual or others
2. An increasing sense of arousal or tension prior to committing or engaging in the act
3. An experience of either pleasure, gratification, or release of tension at the time of committing the act.

In addition, there is usually a pattern of engaging in the abnormal behavior in spite of adverse consequences (e.g., criminal charges, impairment of normal functioning, etc.).

There are several discrete categories of impulse control disorders defined in DSM-III-R. *Intermittent explosive disorder* is diagnosed when an individual displays episodic loss of control of aggressive impulses without signs of generalized impulsivity or aggressivity. There is some debate about the validity of this disorder (Monopolis and Lion 1983), however, and it is possible that it will not be included as a distinct diagnostic entity in DSM-IV (Wise 1990). In *pyromania* there is impulsive, repetitive, deliberate fire setting without external reward (e.g., arson for money, revenge, as a political act). In addition, fire setting may be seen in a wide variety of psychiatric disorders (Geller 1987). *Kleptomania* is a disorder in which the individual impulsively steals even though there is no need to do so (i.e., the individual has money to pay for the stolen items or does not need the stolen goods). *Pathological gambling* is diagnosed when there is a failure to resist impulses to gamble that interferes with social and occupational functioning (see Chapter 8). *Trichotillomania* is a disorder in which there are irresistible impulses for the individual to pull out his or her own hair (see Chapter 5). There have also been proposals to include other disorders of impulse control in this diagnostic class (e.g., repetitive self-mutilation disorder, compulsive shopping; see Wise 1990).

Other Axis I disorders such as the paraphilias, bulimia, and substance use disorders also involve an inability to resist harmful impulses, a sense of arousal or tension prior to engaging in the pathological behavior, and the experience of pleasure and release of tension afterward. Consequently, these may also be considered disorders of impulse control.

In contrast to the episodic loss of impulse control found in the Axis I disorders described above, chronic aggressive or impulsive behavior is often characteristic of individuals with personality disorders, especially borderline personality disorder (BPD) and antisocial personality disorder. Three of the eight criteria for BPD in DSM-III-R describe types of impulsive aggressive behavior: a) impulsiveness in at least two areas that are potentially self-damaging (e.g., spending, sex, substance use, shoplifting, reckless driving, binge eating); b) inappropriate, intense anger or lack of control of anger; and c) recurrent suicidal threats, gestures, or behavior, or self-mutilating behavior. Similarly, the criteria for antisocial personality disorder also include manifestations of impulse dyscontrol: a person with this disorder a) is irritable and aggressive, as indicated by repeated physical fights or assaults; b) shows failure to plan ahead, or is impulsive; and c) has reckless regard of his or her own or others' personal safety (e.g., driving while intoxicated or recurrent speeding).

Consequently, there is wide diagnostic overlap among disorders of impulse control. For example, the criteria for BPD contain impulsive behaviors such as kleptomania, binge eating, and substance abuse. Accordingly, a more parsimonious perspective may be one in which personality psychopathology such as impulsivity and/or aggressivity is viewed within a dimensional, rather than categorical, model (Widiger et al. 1987; also see Chapter 12).

Family History

There are few family history studies of specific impulse control disorders. However, an increased prevalence of impulse dyscontrol (i.e., manifested by episodic temper outbursts) in first-degree relatives of psychiatric patients with temper outbursts, compared with similar patients without this history, has been reported (18% versus 4%, respectively; Mattes and Fink 1987). Moreover, history of temper outbursts, as a discrete and uncomplicated behavioral variable, displayed greater familial aggregation than did specific psychiatric diagnosis (e.g., intermittent explosive disorder, BPD/antisocial personality disorder, or attention-deficit disorder—residual); increased familial aggregation of temper outbursts was not observed in patients with neurological conditions.

In addition, family history studies suggest a relationship between impulse control disorders and affective disorders and/or substance abuse. In one study (Linden et al. 1986), first-degree relatives of compulsive gamblers displayed an increased prevalence of affective disorders and alcohol abuse (76% and 36%, respectively). In another study, violent offenders and impulsive fire setters also had an elevated prevalence of alcoholism. Moreover, violent offenders and impulsive fire setters with alcoholic fathers had lower mean cerebrospinal (CSF) 5-hydroxyindoleacetic acid (5-HIAA) concentrations and were more impulsive than were similar subjects without alcoholic fathers (Linnoila et al. 1989), raising the possibility that impulse dyscontrol, alcoholism, and reduced central serotonergic system function may be coinherited. Further evidence of this possibility is suggested by the observation of a familial aggregation of impulsive personality disorder traits (and possibly of affective personality and alcoholism) in males with personality disorders who have reduced prolactin responses to fenfluramine challenge (Coccaro et al. 1991b).

Etiology

The causes of aggressivity and/or impulsivity are multidetermined. Aggressive or violent behavior is often volitional and not the result of psychiatric disturbance. Impulsivity is common in psychiatric disorders that are associated with impaired judgment: psychosis, organic mental disorders (e.g., organic personality disorder, temporal lobe epilepsy), and mood disorders (e.g., bipolar disorder—manic). In addition, acting-out behavior may be used as a form of communication by an individual with impaired interpersonal skills. Social and cultural factors also play an important role in this regard, although a full discussion of this topic is beyond the scope of this chapter. Finally, there is evidence that certain impulsive aggressive behaviors may be predetermined by dynamic, behavioral, and biological factors.

Many psychoanalytic hypotheses of impulse dyscontrol have not been empirically tested. Acting out of impulses has often been seen as an expression of the need to express an unacceptable sexual or aggressive drive. For example, Freud (1933[1932]/1964) equated the sensations associated with setting fires to sexual excitement. In compulsive gambling there may be an unconscious need to lose and experience punishment for unconscious aggression (Bergler 1957).

An intriguing behavioral model of self-destructive behavior in BPD, specifically, has been postulated by Linehan (1987). This model proposes that innate deficits in affective regulation are coupled with an environment in which these abnormal affects are not validated. In turn, the individual does not learn the skills needed to regulate these affects and instead acts out or turns to self-destructive behavior. This model, however, awaits empirical validation.

Biological systems have been suggested to play a role in the development of impulsive aggressive behaviors. First, an association between abnormal platelet monoamine oxidase (MAO) activity (a putative measure of central monoaminergic function) and "impulsive" and "sensation-seeking" personality traits has been reported, regardless of specific psychiatric diagnosis, in at least two studies (Buchsbaum et al. 1976; Zuckerman et al. 1980). Reduced platelet MAO activity correlated with self-rated impulsivity in depressed male patients in another study (Perris et al. 1984). Similarly, reduced platelet MAO activity in males with BPD, when compared with that of healthy volunteers, was reported in two other studies (Reist et al. 1990; Yehuda et al. 1989). Finally, inverse relationships between platelet MAO activity and sensation seeking in male BPD patients (Reist et al. 1990), as well as between verbal hostility and trait impulsivity in female BPD patients (Soloff et al. 1991), have also been reported.

Overall, however, the most widely studied neurotransmitter system in regard to impulsive and/or aggressive behavior is the central serotonergic system. Associations between indices of central serotonergic system dysfunction and indices of impulsivity and/or aggressivity have been reported widely in mammalian species (including humans) for nearly two decades.

Animal studies have consistently demonstrated an inverse relationship between aggressive responding and central serotonergic system function. In rats, for example, p-chlorophenylalanine, a serotonin (5-hydroxytryptamine [5-HT]) synthesis inhibitor, increases aggressive behavior. Similarly, shock-induced fighting in rats is potentiated by pretreatment with the 5-HT neuronal toxin 5,7-dihydroxytryptamine (Kantak et al. 1981). Conversely, 5-hydroxytryptophan (a 5-HT precursor) reverses aggressive behavior associated with the lesioning of the 5-HT–rich olfactory bulbs (Dichiara et al. 1971). Also, mouse-killing behavior following pretreatment with p-chlorophenylalanine is blocked by the 5-HT reuptake inhibitor fluoxetine (Berzenyi et al. 1983).

Studies of serotonin functioning in humans have also demonstrated a relationship with impulsivity and/or aggressivity. The first to suggest this relationship were Åsberg et al. (1976), who demonstrated an association between reduced CSF 5-HIAA concentration and violent suicidal behavior in depressed patients. Subsequently, Brown et al. (1979) found an inverse relationship between life history of physical aggression and CSF 5-HIAA concentration in military recruits with DSM-II personality disorders. Many, though not all, studies report inverse correlations between CSF 5-HIAA concentration and impulsive behavior in humans, regardless of specific psychiatric diagnosis (Brown and Linnoila 1990; Coccaro 1989). For example, violent offenders and impulsive fire setters with a history of serious suicide attempts (i.e., requiring hospital admission) were found to have lower CSF 5-HIAA concentrations than similar subjects without history of serious suidical behavior (Virkunnen et al. 1987).

Reduced CSF 5-HIAA concentration in these individuals was further associated with future violent acts or impulsive fire setting during a follow-up period of 3 years.

These findings have not been limited to adults. CSF 5-HIAA concentrations measured in children and adolescents with disruptive behavior disorders (i.e., attention-deficit disorder, oppositional disorder, and conduct disorder) were inversely correlated with measures of aggressivity but not those of impulsivity (Kruesi et al. 1990). CSF 5-HIAA concentration has also been inversely correlated with history of cruelty to animals in children (Kruesi 1989).

Reduced CSF 5-HIAA concentration appears to correlate specifically with impulsive, rather than premeditated, aggression (Linnoila et al. 1983). Similarly, impulsive fire setters (i.e., pyromaniacs) demonstrate lower CSF 5-HIAA concentrations than do fire setters who also engage in other, nonimpulsive antisocial acts (Virkkunen et al. 1987). This finding suggests that indices of central serotonergic system function correlate more specifically with overt impulsive behaviors than with covert nonimpulsive (e.g., conning) behaviors.

Depressed patients with reduced CSF 5-HIAA concentrations show not only an increased rate of suicide attempts but also an increased frequency of outwardly directed aggression (van Praag 1986). In addition, CSF 5-HIAA concentrations correlate inversely with suicidal behavior (i.e., suicide attempts) in schizophrenic individuals (Ninan et al. 1984; van Praag 1983), and with outwardly directed hostility (e.g., irritability) in healthy volunteers without a psychiatric diagnosis (Roy et al. 1988a). These findings suggest that abnormalities in central serotonergic system function may be associated with impulsive aggressive behavior as a personality dimension regardless of either psychiatric diagnosis or direction of aggression.

Pharmacochallenge studies in which the neuroendocrine and/or behavioral response to acute challenge with specific serotonergic agents is examined have also demonstrated evidence of a relationship between central serotonergic system function and impulsive aggression. One advantage of this method is that the outcome measures tend to reflect dynamic indices of central serotonergic systems, perhaps in specific brain areas (e.g., within the limbic-hypothalamic-pituitary axis).

To date, there have been several pharmacochallenge studies examining impulsivity and/or aggressivity directly. The first reported a strong inverse relationship between the prolactin response to fenfluramine challenge and indices of irritable, impulsive aggression in male patients with personality disorders regardless of categorical distinctions such as the presence of BPD or a past history of suicidal or alcohol-abusing behavior (Coccaro et al. 1989b). Although another study of alcohol- and substance-abusing patients suggests a direct relationship between these two variables (Fishbein et al. 1989), other data are consistent with an inverse relationship between indices of central serotonergic system function and of impulsive aggression in patients with mood and/or personality disorders. These data were derived utilizing fenfluramine (DeMeo et al. 1989) or direct 5-HT receptor agonist probes such as the 5-HT_1–like agent *m*-chlorophenylpiperazine (Coccaro et al. 1989a; Hollander et al. 1990; Moss et al. 1990) or the 5-HT_{1A}–like agent buspirone (Coccaro et al. 1990b).

Other measures of central serotonergic system function are also abnormal in patients with a history of aggressive behavior. In postmortem studies, tritiated imipramine binding (a presynaptic 5-HT index) is reduced in the brains of violent suicide victims (Stanley et al. 1982). Similarly, indices of 5-HT platelet uptake correlate inversely with indices of impulsivity in male patients with episodic aggression (Brown et al. 1989). In addition, 5-HT platelet uptake is reduced in impulsive alcohol abusers (Bailly et al. 1990). Conversely, indices of increased postsynaptic 5-HT_2 receptor binding in the prefrontal cortex of brain of suicide victims (Arango et al. 1990; Mann et al. 1986), especially those using violent methods (Arora and Meltzer 1989), have been reported. While this may represent a compensatory response within the central serotonergic system, it is possible that this reflects an independent abnormality in the central serotonergic system (Coccaro 1989).

Disturbances of catecholaminergic functioning in impulse dyscontrol disorders may also be present. Dopaminergic (Pucilowski et al. 1986) and adrenergic (Kantak et al. 1981) manipulations have been found to affect aggression in rats in a direct fashion. Several studies have compared adrenergic and noradrenergic receptor binding in brain of suicide completers with those in brain of accident victims.

Consistent with animal data, increased ß-adrenergic receptor binding in the prefrontal/temporal cortex is reported in suicide completers in many (Arango et al. 1990; Biegon and Israeli 1988; Mann et al. 1986), though not all (Stockmeier and Meltzer 1991), studies. Conversely, reduced α_1-noradrenegic receptor binding has been reported in the prefrontal/temporal cortex and in the caudate nucleus of suicide completers (Gross-Isseroff et al. 1990). Similarly, a decrease in platelet α_2-noradrenergic high-affinity binding sites was reported in BPD patients compared with healthy volunteers and depressed patients (Southwick et al. 1990). However, because the reduction in binding sites was confined to unmedicated BPD patients, it is possible that this abnormality is related more specifically to anxiety rather than to personality traits such as impulsivity.

Cerebrospinal fluid and pharmacochallenge studies in impulse dyscontrol patients provide findings that are more consistent with a direct role of noradrenergic system function. Specifically, higher, rather than lower, CSF 3-methoxy-4-hydroxyphenylglycol (MHPG) and urinary norepinephrine concentrations have been reported in pathological gamblers compared with healthy volunteers (Roy et al. 1988b). Strong positive correlations were also noted between these indices of central noradrenergic system function and indices of "extraversion" (Roy et al. 1989). These findings suggest that an abnormality in central noradrenergic system function may underlie the sensation-seeking characteristic of the compulsive gambler. Similarly, urinary norepinephrine concentrations were higher in depressed patients with a history of suicidal behavior compared with depressed patients without this history in one study in which elevated urinary norepinephrine concentrations were correlated with low suicidal intent (i.e., impulsivity) (Brown and Mancini 1991). Finally, a direct correlation between irritability (but not assaultiveness) and growth hormone response to the α_2-adrenoceptor agonist clonidine has been observed in male patients with personality disorders and in healthy male volunteers (Coccaro et al. 1991a). Curiously, two of these studies suggest no relationship between indices of noradrenergic and serotonergic system function (Coccaro et al. 1991a; Roy et al. 1989) raising the possibility that the influences of these two neuronal systems on behaviors related to irritable impulsiveness are independent.

Treatment

Psychodynamic treatment modalities for impulse control disorders (especially impulsive/acting-out personality disorders) have been widely discussed in the literature. Both supportive psychotherapy and intensive analytic psychotherapy have been advocated for the treatment of these patients (Aronson 1989). Intensive, restructuring therapies seek to help the patient overcome difficulties encountered in the separation-individuation stage of psychic development (Kernberg 1984). Supportive approaches involve reinforcement rather than analysis of psychic defenses, strict limit setting, structured sessions, and establishment of real emotional contact (e.g., acting like a real person) rather than fostering regression (Zetzel 1971). Unfortunately there has been little empirical evidence for the effectiveness of these treatment modalities. Moreover, some investigators suggest that no treatment may be indicated for patients with severe oppositional, pervasively impulsive, antisocial personalities (Frances et al. 1984).

Most behavioral treatments for impulse control disorders have used aversive techniques with little empirical evidence of efficacy. Linehan (1987), however, has devised an innovative behavioral treatment program for self-destructive patients. This treatment is structured and directed toward teaching the patient various skills to deal with, and to tolerate, rapidly shifting, intense affective states. This approach uses instruction, modeling, behavioral and cognitive rehearsal, cognitive restructuring, and operant conditioning (i.e., reinforcement). Empirical trials to determine the efficacy of this treatment are ongoing.

Given our rapidly expanding knowledge of the biological bases of impulsivity and aggressivity, there is widening interest in the use of psychopharmacological agents to treat disorders of impulse control. To date, most reports regarding the psychopharmacological treatment of impulse dyscontrol have been uncontrolled case studies. However there have been some controlled studies regarding the pharmacotherapy of impulsive (i.e., borderline) personality disorders that may be helpful in devising treatment strategies for other patients with impulse dyscontrol. The medications most widely studied include neuroleptic and antidepressant agents, lithium, carbamaze-pine, benzodiazepines, ß-noradrenergic receptor antagonists, and 5-HT reuptake blockers and agonists.

Neuroleptic agents have been widely used to treat impulsive aggressive behavior. However, it is not clear whether the antiaggres-sive effects of these agents are related to dopaminergic blockade or to nonspecific sedation. Open-label thioridazine has been reported to diminish impulse action (e.g., as gauged by the Diagnostic Interview for Borderlines) in patients with BPD as well as in ratings related to psychosis (Teicher et al. 1989). Similarly, treatment with low-dose haloperidol was associated with significant improvement in ratings of hostility, impulsivity, depression, and schizotypal symp-toms, compared with amitriptyline and placebo, in a large sample of patients with BPD and/or schizotypal personality disorder. This observation was not apparent, however, in two other double-blind, placebo-controlled studies of BPD and/or schizotypal personality disorder patients treated with thiothixene (Goldberg et al. 1986) or trifluoperazine (Cowdry and Gardner 1988). On the other hand, flupentixol significantly reduced suicidal behavior in a placebo-con-trolled study of personality disorder patients with a history of multiple impulsive suicide attempts (Montgomery and Montgomery 1982). This finding suggests that low-dose neuroleptic agents may be an effective treatment for selected patients with impulse dyscontrol. Regardless, the risk of extrapyramidal side effects such as akathisia and tardive dyskinesia warrants caution in the indiscriminate use of these agents in patients with impulse control problems.

A putative link between impulsivity/aggressivity and mood and anxiety disorders (Apter et al. 1990) suggests that antidepressant medications might be efficacious in treating impulse dyscontrol. Unfortunately, tricyclic antidepressants have been associated with increased impulse dyscontrol in subgroups of personality disorder patients, particularly those patients prone to impulse dyscontrol (Soloff et al. 1986). In one well-designed study, amitriptyline was generally less effective than haloperidol in this regard (Soloff et al. 1989); almost half of the amitriptyline-treated patients had more acting-out behavior than at baseline. Moreover, efficacy of the tricyclic appeared to be confined to depressive symptoms, with presence of paranoia and schizotypy associated with poorer out-come. In another double-blind study, desipramine was no better than placebo in treating patients with BPD (Links et al. 1990). MAO inhibitors yield variable therapeutic results in patients with impulsive personality disorders. Improvement in mood was reported in one study of BPD patients treated with tranylcypromine, compared with carbamazepine, trifluoperazine, alprazolam, or placebo (Cowdry and Gardner 1988). Improvement in impulse control, however, was only apparent on self-report ratings. Similarly, global response was greater for phenelzine than for imipramine in a second study of atypically depressed patients with BPD (Parsons et al. 1989). On the other hand, the most recent study of MAO inhibitor agents reports little therapeu-tic benefit to using these agents in BPD patients (Cornelius et al. 1991).

A positive effect of benzodiazepine-like agents in patients with impulsive personality disorders has been reported for alprazolam in BPD patients (Faltus 1984). However, recent evidence suggests that these agents may actually increase impulse dyscontrol in these individuals (Dietch and Jennings 1988). Specifically, Cowdry and Gardner (1988) reported that alprazolam, compared with placebo, increased the frequency of behavioral dyscontrol in BPD patients. Thus, these agents should be used with caution in this population.

Beta-adrenergic receptor antagonists have been used effectively to treat aggressive behavior in certain psychiatric populations, al-though the studies have not been controlled and the mechanism of action is unclear. High doses of propranolol may decrease aggressive behavior in various patients with chronic organic brain syndromes (Yudofsky et al. 1981), in patients with schizophrenia (Sorgi et al. 1986), or in adults with temper outbursts and residual attention-deficit disorder (Mattes 1986). Further controlled studies are needed in patients with impulse control disorders and personality disorders.

Lithium carbonate may also be of value in the treatment of patients with impulse control disorders. Lithium was more effective than placebo in reducing mood lability in patients with "emotionally unstable character disorder" (Rifkin et al. 1972), a diagnostic category similar to BPD, characterized by intense, rapidly shifting affects and variably associated with impulse dyscontrol. Lithium was also superior to desipramine and placebo in BPD patients on indices of global behavior (Links et al. 1990). More important, lithium has been reported to reduce impulsive aggression in prison inmates in both open (Tupin et al. 1973) and blind placebo-controlled trials (Sheard et al. 1976) and in blind placebo-contolled trials in hospitalized children with conduct disorder (Campbell et al. 1984). Case reports also suggest the efficacy of lithium in specific impulse control disorders such as compulsive gambling (Moskowitz 1980) and tricho-tillomania (Christenson et al. 1991). Although the exact mechanism of lithium's efficacy in impulsive disorders is unknown, it may be due to lithium's ability to enhance serotonergic, and/or to diminish catecholaminergic, transmission (Bunney and Garland-Bunney 1987).

Carbamazepine, an anticonvulsant, is another agent that may be efficacious in the treatment of impulse control disorders and impulsive personalities. Open-label trials with carbamazepine suggest that this agent may be effective in reducing self-destructive behavior in patients with mental retardation (Winchel and Stanley 1991). One blind, placebo-controlled trial found carbamazepine to be the only agent that selectively decreased behavioral dyscontrol (Cowdry and Gardner 1988). Although the exact mechanism of action is unclear, carbamazepine has been reported to increase plasma levels of the 5-HT precursor tryptophan (Pratt et al. 1984), and to increase the prolactin response to tryptophan challenge (Elphick et al. 1990). This finding raises the possibility of a central serotonergic mode of action for carbamazepine.

The effect of central serotonergic agents on impulse dyscontrol has, despite a compelling rationale, received only limited study to date. Open treatment with 5-hydroxytryptophan (a 5-HT precursor) to self-injuring patients with Lesch-Nyhan syndrome decreased self-injurious behavior in one study (Mizuno and Yugari 1974). Similarly, in another study, self-injurious behavior in patients with coexisting OCD responded to treatment with serotonergic agents (Primeau and Fontaine 1987). Self-injury in a patient with major depression also responded to trazodone (Patel et al. 1988), a medication with both 5-HT agonist and antagonistic properties. The 5-HT uptake inhibitor clomipramine was effective in reducing hair-pulling behavior in trichotillomanic patients in an open trial (Pollard et al. 1991) and was more effective than desipramine in reducing this behavior in a double-blind study (Swedo et al. 1989). Finally, three patients with comorbid kleptomania and bulimia nervosa responded to fluoxetine, trazodone, or tranylcypromine, all of which appear to act through serotonergic mechanisms (McElroy et al. 1989).

Studies with serotonergic agents in patients with personality disorders are only in their beginning stages. The 5-HT–specific reuptake inhibitor fluoxetine was reported to be generally efficacious during open-label treatment in some BPD patients, particularly those without comorbid depression (Norden 1989). Similar responses to open-label fluoxetine were reported in inpatient BPD patients, especially in regard to suicidal ideation and impulse dyscontrol, though not with respect to interpersonal sensitivity (Cornelius et al. 1990). In another open-label study, fluoxetine treatment was specifically associated with substantial reductions in overt aggressive behavior and irritability in three nondepressed personality disorder outpatients with histories of prominent impulsive aggressive behavior (Coccaro et al. 1990a). On the other hand, some anecdotal reports suggest that fluoxetine may be associated with an increase in suicidal and/or aggressive behavior in rare cases (Teicher et al. 1990). These observations are controversial, however, and data from a more recent placebo-controlled study of fluoxetine in personality diosorder patients with recurrent suicidal behavior do not support this observation (Montgomery and Montgomery 1991). Other 5-HT reuptake blockers (e.g., paroxetine, sertraline, fluvoxamine) may also prove effective in reduction of aggressive behavior. 5-HT$_1$–like agonists may also be effective, although one recent double-blind, placebo-controlled study of the incomplete 5-HT$_{1A}$ agonist buspirone reported no efficacy for this agent in BPD patients (Wolf et al. 1991). Whether this will also be true for full 5-HT$_1$–like agonists such as gepirone, ipsapirone, or eltoprazine remains for further study.

Methodological Problems

There are several methodological problems with the studies of impulse control and aggressive disorders in humans conducted to date. One problem relates to the definition of impulsivity. It is often difficult to distinguish impulsive behavior from volitional behavior or from behavior motivated by external factors. Episodic impulsivity and circumscribed impulsivity (e.g., stealing, excessive gambling, fire setting) often occur along with impulsive personality disorders, making it difficult to study Axis I and Axis II disorders separately. It is also difficult, though important, to distinguish among impulsivity, irritability, sensation seeking, and aggressive behaviors in order to correlate the behavior of interest with appropriate psychosocial factors, biological and genetic markers, and treatment strategies.

The influence of drugs and alcohol must also be considered in future studies. These substances reduce impulse control but may also be self-administered by the patient in his or her attempt to deal with overwhelming, intense impulses. Thus, some substance abusers may be "self-treating" their underlying impulse dyscontrol with agents that may acutely, though only temporarily, act like some potentially therapeutic agents (Ballenger et al. 1979).

Also posing difficulties in this regard is the fact that impulsive behaviors and aggressive outbursts are usually of short duration and of varying frequency. Thus, it is difficult to distinguish possible state and trait biological indices for impulsivity. It is especially difficult to carry out treatment trials with this population because the base rate of behavior can fluctuate so markedly. Future studies must include longer initial and treatment response assessment periods, double-blind discontinuation studies, and long-term follow-up.

Aggressive and impulsive behaviors are often associated with a wide range of social factors (see above), and yet these factors have not been fully explored in relation to studies of biological markers and medication treatment of the impulse control disorders. Future studies will need to explore the relationship between psychosocial factors and biological markers in these disorders. For example, impulse control disorders may be associated with an abnormality in serotonergic regulation, with the exact nature of the impulsive behavior (e.g., drinking, gambling, fire setting) determined by behavioral, psychodynamic, family systems, and/or cultural factors.

Another major problem in studies conducted to date is that biological indices may be more closely related to dimensions of behavior than to discrete nosologic categories (Coccaro et al. 1989b; Siever et al. 1985). For example, phenomenologic indices for aggression, anxiety, depression, and suicidality are correlated with each other and appear to be related to abnormalities in serotonergic functioning (Apter et al. 1990). Unfortunately, most previous medication trials in these disorders have selected patients for participation based on categorical diagnosis (e.g., borderline personality) rather than for traits of impulsivity and/or aggressivity. Future psychopharmacological treatment trials in impulse disorders should select patients based on trait impulsivity and/or aggressivity rather than on current nosologic categories. Because biological indices of central serotonergic system function correlate with this dimension of behavior, clinical treatment trials should strive, whenever possible, to correlate treatment responsiveness with biological indices.

Relationship of Impulse Control Disorders to Obsessive-Compulsive Disorder

There are interesting similarities in the phenomenology, biology, and treatment response between OCD and disorders of impulse control. Common to both OCD and the impulse control disorders are intrusive, irresistible urges to commit an act that may or may not be seen as senseless. In addition, many patients with either disorder experience a mounting tension associated with attempts to resist the behavior, and relief from anxiety following their engagement in the behavior.

Based upon the evidence reviewed in this chapter, there is a clear relationship between central serotonergic system function and impulsive aggressive behavior. This relationship does not appear to be specific for any one categorical psychiatric diagnosis. Moreover, abnormalities in central serotonergic system function are also reported in patients with OCD. For example, OCD patients appear to be behaviorally hyperresponsive to administration of central 5-HT agonists (Hollander et al. 1988, 1992; Zohar et al. 1987). In addition, 5-HT reuptake blockers appear to be more efficacious in OCD compared with nonselective antidepressants (Goodman et al. 1990).

It is possible that serotonin acts as a neurochemical inhibitor of the expression of various behaviors. Hence, it is tempting to conceptualize impulsive and compulsive behavior as occurring on opposite ends of a continuum of behavior modulated by serotonin (e.g., too much 5-HT activity inhibiting behavior in OCD; too little 5-HT activity to inhibit impulsive acts in patients with impulse dyscontrol). Undoubtedly, however, this model is as oversimplistic as those positing that depression and panic disorders result simply from too little or too much central noradrenergic system function, respectively. Accordingly, as human behaviors are probably influenced by the interaction of multiple transmitter systems (Coccaro and Murphy 1990), further investigations will be required before the relationship between impulsive and compulsive behavior is clarified.

Conclusions

The impulsive personality disorders and Axis I disorders of impulse control are a superficially heterogeneous group of disorders that may share a common underlying biological basis and respond to similar biological and psychosocial treatment interventions. These disorders also appear to share features with OCD in terms of phenomenology, biology, and treatment response. Future studies must correlate dimensions of psychopathology such as impulsivity/aggressivity with biological indices rather than with currently available categorical diagnoses. Finally, as we become more sophisticated in our ability to measure biological indices associated with various dimensions of psychopathology, it will be further important to correlate responses to psychopharmacological treatment with relevant biological indices.

References

American Psychiatric Association: Diagnostic and Statistical Manual of Mental Disorders, 3rd Edition. Washington, DC, American Psychiatric Association, 1980

American Psychiatric Association: Diagnostic and Statistical Manual of Mental Disorders, 3rd Edition, Revised. Washington, DC, American Psychiatric Association, 1987

Apter A, van Praag HM, Plutchik R, et al: Interrelationships among anxiety, aggression, impulsivity, and mood: a serotonergically linked cluster? Psychiatry Res 32:191–199, 1990

Arango V, Ernsberger P, Marzuk PM, et al: Autoradiographic demonstration of increased serotonin 5HT2 and 1-adrenergic receptor binding sites in the brain of suicide victims. Arch Gen Psychiatry 47:1038–1047, 1990

Aronson TA: A critical review of psychotherapeutic treatments of the borderline personality: historical trends and future directions. J Nerv Ment Dis 177:511–528, 1989

Arora RC, Meltzer HY: Serotonergic measures in the brains of suicide victims: 5HT2 binding sites in the frontal cortex of suicide victims and control subjects. Am J Psychiatry 146:730–736, 1989

Åsberg M, Träskman L, Thorén P: 5-HIAA in the cerebrospinal fluid: a biochemical suicide predictor? Arch Gen Psychiatry 33:1193–1197, 1976

Bailly D, Vignau J, Lauth B, et al: Platelet serotonin decrease in alcoholic patients. Acta Psychiatr Scand 81:68–72, 1990

Ballenger JC, Goodwin FK, Major LF, et al: Alcohol and central serotonin metabolism in man. Arch Gen Psychiatry 36:224–227, 1979

Bergler E: The Psychology of Gambling. New York, International Universities Press, 1957

Berzenyi P, Galateo E, Valzelli L: Fluoxetine activity on muricidal aggression induced in rats by p-chlorophenylalanine. Aggressive Behavior 9:333–338, 1983

Biegon A, Israeli M: Regionally selective increases in beta-adrenergic receptor density in brains of suicide victims. Brain Res 442:199–203, 1988

Brown CS, Kent TA, Bryant SG, et al: Blood platelet uptake of serotonin in episodic aggression. Psychiatry Res 27:5–12, 1989

Brown G, Mancini C: Urinary catecholamines and cortisol in suicide, in New Research Program and Abstracts, 144th annual meeting of the American Psychiatric Association, New Orleans, LA, May 1991, NR660, p 206

Brown GL, Linnoila MI: CSF serotonin metabolite (5-HIAA) studies in depression, impulsivity, and violence. J Clin Psychiatry 51 (no 4, suppl):31–41,1990

Brown GL, Goodwin FK, Ballenger JC, et al: Aggression in humans correlates with cerebrospinal fluid metabolite. Psychiatry Res 1:131–139, 1979

Buchsbaum MS, Coursey RD, Murphy DL: The biochemical high risk paradigm: behavioral and familial correlates of low platelet monoamine oxidase activity. Science 194:339–341, 1976

Bunney WE Jr, Garland-Bunney BL: Mechanisms of action of lithium in affective illness: basic and clinical implications, in Psychopharmacology: The Third Generation of Progress. Edited by Meltzer HY. New York, Raven, 1987, pp 553–565

Campbell M, Small AM, Green WH, et al: Behavioral efficacy of haloperidol and lithium carbonate: a comparison in hospitalized aggressive children with conduct disorder. Arch Gen Psychiatry 41:650–656, 1984

Christenson GA, Popkin MK, Mackenzie TB, et al: Lithium treatment of chronic hair pulling. J Clin Psychiatry 52:116–120, 1991

Coccaro EF: Central serotonin and impulsive aggression. Br J Psychiatry 155 (suppl 8):52–62, 1989

Coccaro EF, Murphy DL (eds): Serotonin in Major Psychiatric Disorders. Washington, DC, American Psychiatric Press, 1990

Coccaro EF, Siever LJ, Kavoussi R, et al: Impulsive aggression in personality disorder: evidence for involvement of 5-HT-1 receptors. Biol Psychiatry 25:86A, 1989a

Coccaro EF, Siever LJ, Klar HM, et al: Serotonergic studies in patients with affective and personality disorders: correlations with suicidal and impulsive aggressive behavior. Arch Gen Psychiatry 46:587–599, 1989b

Coccaro EF, Astill JL, Herbert JL, et al: Fluoxetine treatment of impulsive aggression in DSM-III-R personality disorder patients (letter). J Clin Psychopharmacol 10:373–375, 1990a

Coccaro EF, Gabriel S, Siever LJ: Buspirone challenge: preliminary evidence for a role for central 5HT$_{1a}$ receptor function in impulsive aggressive behavior in humans. Psychopharmacol Bull 26:393–405, 1990b

Coccaro EF, Lawrence T, Trestman R, et al: Growth hormone responses to intravenous clonidine challenge correlate with behavioral irritability in psychiatric patients and healthy volunteers. Psychiatry Res 39:129–139, 1991a

Coccaro EF, Silverman JM, Klar HM, et al: Familial correlates of reduced central 5-HT function in DSM-III personality disorder patients. Biol Psychiatry 29:97A, 1991b

Cornelius JR, Soloff PH, Perel JM, et al: Fluoxetine trial in borderline personality disorder. Psychopharmacol Bull 26:151–154, 1990

Cornelius JR, Soloff PH, George AW, et al: Phenelzine versus haloperidol in borderline personality, in New Research Program and Abstracts, 144th annual meeting of the American Psychiatric Association, New Orleans, LA, May 1991, NR580, p 188

Cowdry RW, Gardner DL: Pharmacotherapy of borderline personality disorder: alprazolam, carbamazepine, trifluoperazine, and tranylcypromine. Arch Gen Psychiatry 45:111–119, 1988

DeMeo MD, McBride PA, Chen J-S, et al: Relative contribution of MDD and borderline personality disorder to 5-HT responsivity. Biol Psychiatry 25:85A, 1989

Dichiara G, Camba R, Spano PF: Evidence for inhibition by brain serotonin of mouse killing behavior in rats. Nature 233:272–273, 1971

Dietch JT, Jennings RK: Aggressive dyscontrol in patients treated with benzodiazepines. J Clin Psychiatry 49:184–188, 1988

Elphick M, Yang JD, Cowen PJ: Effects of carbamazepine on dopamine- and serotonin-mediated neuroendocrine responses. Arch Gen Psychiatry 47:135–140, 1990

Faltus FJ: The positive effect of alprazolam in the treatment of three patients with borderline personality disorder. Am J Psychiatry 141:802–803, 1984

Fishbein DH, Lozovsky D, Jaffe JH: Impulsivity, aggression, and neuroendocrine responses to serotonergic stimulation in substance abusers. Biol Psychiatry 25:1049–1066, 1989

Frances A, Clarkin J, Perry S: Differential Therapeutics in Psychiatry: The Art and Science of Treatment Selection. New York, Brunner/Mazel, 1984

Freud S: New introductory lectures on psycho-analysis (1933[1932]), in The Standard Edition of the Complete Psychological Works of Sigmund Freud, Vol 22. Translated and edited by Strachey J. London, Hogarth, 1964, pp 1–182

Geller JL: Firesetting in the adult psychiatric population. Hosp Community Psychiatry 38:501–506, 1987

Goldberg SC, Schulz SC, Schulz PM, et al: Borderline and schizotypal personality disorders treated with low-dose thiothixene versus placebo. Arch Gen Psychiatry 43:680–686, 1986

Goodman WK, Price LH, Delgado PL, et al: Specificity of serotonin reuptake inhibitors in the treatment of obsessive-compulsive disorder: comparison of fluvoxamine and desipramine. Arch Gen Psychiatry 47:577–585, 1990

Gross-Isseroff R, Dillon KA, Fieldust SJ, et al: Autoradiographic analysis of 1-noradrenergic receptors in the human brain postmortem: effect of suicide. Arch Gen Psychiatry 47:1049–1053, 1990

Hollander E, Fay M, Cohen B, et al: Serotonergic and noradrenergic sensitivity in obsessive-compulsive disorder: behavioral findings. Am J Psychiatry 145:1015–1017, 1988

Hollander E, DeCaria C, Kellman D, et al: Serotonergic and neuropsychiatric function in impulsive personality disorders. Biol Psychiatry 27:163A, 1990

Hollander E, DeCaria C, Nitescua A, et al: Serotonergic function in obsessive-compulsive disorder: behavioral and neuroendocrine responses to oral m-chlorophenylpiperazine and fenfluramine in patients and healthy volunteers. Arch Gen Psychiatry 49:21–28, 1992

Kantak KM, Hegstrand LR, Eichelman BR: Facilitation of shock-induced fighting following intraventricular 5,7-hydroxytryptamine and 6-hydroxydopa. Psychopharmacology (Berlin) 74:157–160, 1981

Kernberg OF: Severe Personality Disorders: Psychotherapeutic Strategies. New Haven, CT, Yale University Press, 1984

Kruesi MJP: Cruelty to animals and CSF 5HIAA (letter). Psychiatry Res 28:115–116, 1989

Kruesi MJP, Rapoport JL, Hamburger S, et al: Cerebrospinal fluid monoamine metabolites, aggression, and impulsivity in disruptive behavior disorders of children and adolescents. Arch Gen Psychiatry 47:419–426, 1990

Linden RD, Pope HG Jr, Jonas JM: Pathological gambling and major affective disorder: preliminary findings. J Clin Psychiatry 47:201–203, 1986

Linehan MM: Dialectical behavior therapy for borderline personality disorder: theory and method. Bull Menninger Clin 51:261–276, 1987

Links PS, Steiner M, Boiago I, et al: Lithium therapy for borderline patients: preliminary findings. Journal of Personality Disorders 4:173–181, 1990

Linnoila M, Virkkunen M, Scheinin M, et al: Low cerebrospinal fluid 5-hydroxyindoleacetic acid concentration differentiates impulsive from nonimpulsive violent behavior. Life Sci 33:2609–2614, 1983

Linnoila M, De Jong J, Virkkunen M: Family history of alcoholism in violent offenders and impulsive fire setters. Arch Gen Psychiatry 46:613–616, 1989

Mann JJ, Stanley M, McBride PA, et al: Increased serotonin$_2$ and ß-adrenergic receptor binding in frontal cortices of suicide victims. Arch Gen Psychiatry 43:954–959, 1986

Mattes JA: Propranolol for adults with temper outbursts and residual attention deficit disorder. J Clin Psychopharmacol 6:299–302, 1986

Mattes JA, Fink M: A family study of patients with temper outbursts. J Psychiatr Res 21:249–255, 1987

McElroy SL, Keck PE Jr, Pope HG Jr, et al: Pharmacological treatment of kleptomania and bulimia nervosa. J Clin Psychopharmacol 9:358–360, 1989

Mizuno T, Yugari Y: Self-mutilation in Lesch-Nyhan syndrome. Lancet 1:761, 1974

Monopolis S, Lion JR: Problems in the diagnosis of intermittent explosive disorder. Am J Psychiatry 140:1200–1202, 1983

Montgomery SA, Montgomery D: Pharmacological prevention of suicidal behavior. J Affective Disord 4:219–298, 1982

Montgomery D, Montgomery SA: Pharmacotherapy in the prevention of suicidal behavior. Paper presented at the Fourth World Congress of Biological Psychiatry, Florence, Italy, June 1991

Moskowitz JA: Lithium and lady luck: use of lithium carbonate in compulsive gambling. N Y State J Med 80:785–788, 1980

Moss HB, Yao JK, Panzak GL: Serotonergic responsivity and behavioral dimensions in antisocial personality disorder with substance abuse. Biol Psychiatry 28:325–338, 1990

Ninan PT, van Kammen DP, Scheinin M, et al: CSF 5-hydroxyindoleacetic acid levels in suicidal schizophrenic patients. Am J Psychiatry 141:566–569, 1984

Norden MJ: Fluoxetine in borderline personality disorder. Prog Neuropsychopharmacol Biol Psychiatry 13:885–893, 1989

Parsons B, Quitkin FM, McGrath PJ, et al: Phenelzine, imipramine, and placebo in borderline patients meeting criteria for atypical depression. Psychopharmacol Bull 25:524–534, 1989

Patel H, Bruza D, Yeragani VK: Treatment of self-abusive behavior with trazodone (letter). Can J Psychiatry 33:331–332, 1988

Perris C, Eisemann M, Knorring L, et al: Personality traits and monoamine oxidase activity in platelets in depressed patients. Neuropsychobiology 12:201–205, 1984

Pollard CA, Ibe IO, Krojanker DN, et al: Clomipramine treatment of trichotillomania: a follow-up report on four cases. J Clin Psychiatry 52:128–130, 1991

Pratt JA, Jenner P, Johnson AL, et al: Anticonvulsant drugs alter plasma tryptophan concentrations in epileptic patients: implications for antiepileptic action and mental function. J Neurol Neurosurg Psychiatry 47:1131–1133, 1984

Primeau F, Fontaine R: Obsessive disorder with self-mutilation: a subgroup responsive to pharmacotherapy. Can J Psychiatry 32:699–701, 1987

Pucilowski O, Kozak W, Valzelli L: Effect of 6-OHDA injected into the locus coeruleus on apomorphine induced aggression. Pharmacol Biochem Behav 24:773–775, 1986

Reist C, Haier RJ, DeMet E, et al: Platelet MAO activity in personality disorders and normal controls. Psychiatry Res 33:221–227, 1990

Rifkin A, Quitkin F, Carrillo C, et al: Lithium carbonate in emotionally unstable character disorder. Arch Gen Psychiatry 27:519–523, 1972

Roy A, Adinoff B, Linnoila M, et al: Acting out hostility in normal volunteers: negative correlation with levels of 5HIAA in cerebrospinal fluid. Psychiatry Res 24:187–194, 1988a

Roy A, Adinoff B, Roehrich L, et al: Pathological gambling: a psychobiological study. Arch Gen Psychiatry 45:369–373, 1988b

Roy A, De Jong J, Linnoila M: Extraversion in pathological gamblers: correlates with indexes of noradrenergic function. Arch Gen Psychiatry 46:679–681, 1989

Sheard MH, Marini JL, Bridges CI, et al: The effect of lithium on impulsive aggressive behavior in man. Am J Psychiatry 133:1409–1413, 1976

Siever LJ, Klar H, Coccaro E: Psychobiologic substrates of personality, in Biologic Response Styles: Clinical Implications. Edited by Klar H, Siever LJ. Washington, DC, American Psychiatric Press, 1985, pp 37–66

Soloff PH, George A, Nathan RS, et al: Paradoxical effects of amitriptyline on borderline patients. Am J Psychiatry 143:1603–1605, 1986

Soloff PH, George A, Nathan RS, et al: Amitriptyline versus haloperidol in borderlines: final outcomes and predictors of response. J Clin Psychopharmacol 9:238–246, 1989

Soloff PH, Cornelius J, Foglia J, et al: Platelet MAO in borderline personality disorder. Biol Psychiatry 29:499–502, 1991

Sorgi PJ, Ratey JJ, Polakoff S: ß-Adrenergic blockers for the control of aggressive behaviors in patients with chronic schizophrenia. Am J Psychiatry 143:775–776, 1986

Southwick SM, Yehuda R, Giller EL Jr, et al: Altered platelet 2-adrenergic receptor binding sites in borderline personality disorder. Am J Psychiatry 147:1014–1017, 1990

Spitzer RL, Endicott J, Gibbon M: Crossing the border into borderline personality and borderline schizophrenia: the development of criteria. Arch Gen Psychiatry 36:17–24, 1979

Stanley M, Viggilio J, Gershon S: Tritiated imipramine binding sites are decreased in the frontal cortex of suicides. Science 216:1337–1339, 1982

Stockmeier CA, Meltzer HY: ß-Adrenergic receptor binding in the frontal cortex of suicide victims. Biol Psychiatry 29:183–191, 1991

Swedo SE, Leonard HL, Rappoport JL, et al: A double-blind comparison of clomipramine and desipramine in the treatment of trichotillomania. N Engl J Med 321:497–501, 1989

Teicher MH, Glod CA, Aaronson ST, et al: Open assessment of the safety and efficacy of thioridazine in the treatment of patients with borderline personality disorder. Psychopharmacol Bull 25:535–549, 1989

Teicher MH, Glod C, Cole JO: Emergence of intense suicidal preoccupation during fluoxetine treatment. Am J Psychiatry 147:207–210, 1990

Tupin JP, Smith DB, Clanon TL, et al: The long-term use of lithium in aggressive prisoners. Compr Psychiatry 14:311–317, 1973

van Praag HM: CSF 5-HIAA and suicide in non-depressed schizophrenics. Lancet 1:977–978, 1983

van Praag HM: (Auto)aggression and CSF 5-HIAA in depression and schizophrenia. Psychopharmacol Bull 22:669–673, 1986

Virkkunen M, Nuutila A, Goodwin FK, et al: Cerebrospinal fluid monoamine metabolite levels in male arsonists. Arch Gen Psychiatry 44:241–247, 1987

Widiger TA, Trull TJ, Hurt SW, et al: A multidimensional scaling of the DSM-III personality disorders. Arch Gen Psychiatry 44:557–563, 1987

Winchel RM, Stanley M: Self-injurious behavior: a review of the behavior and biology of self-mutilation. Am J Psychiatry 148:306–317, 1991

Wise MG: Impulse control disorders in DSM-IV. American Academy of Psychiatry and Law Newsletter 15:100, 1990

Wolf M, Carreon D, Summers D, et al: Lack of efficacy of buspirone in borderline personality disorder, in New Research Program and Abstracts, 144th annual meeting of the American Psychiatric Association, New Orleans, LA, May 1991, NR302, p 120

Yehuda R, Southwick SM, Edell WS, et al: Low platelet monoamine oxidase activity in borderline personality disorder. Psychiatry Res 30:265–273, 1989

Yudofsky S, Williams D, Gorman J: Propranolol in the treatment of rage and violent behavior in patients with chronic brain syndromes. Am J Psychiatry 138:218–220, 1981

Zetzel ER: A developmental approach to the borderline patient. Am J Psychiatry 127:867–871, 1971

Zohar J, Mueller EA, Insel TR, et al: Serotonergic responsivity in obsessive-compulsive disorder. Arch Gen Psychiatry 44:946–951, 1987

Zuckerman M, Buchsbaum MS, Murphy DL: Sensation seeking and its biological correlates. Psychol Bull 88:187–214, 1980

Chapter 10

Obsessive-Compulsive Symptoms in Schizophrenia

Seth Kindler, M.D.
Zeev Kaplan, M.D.
Joseph Zohar, M.D.

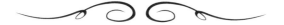

Obsessive-compulsive (OC) symptomatology in schizophrenia, as well as psychotic symptomatology in obsessive-compulsive disorder (OCD) (at one time known as "obsessional neurosis"), has been documented for many years (Robinson et al. 1975; Stengel 1945). The presence of this symptom overlap led some early investigators to conclude that there was a close association between the two disorders (Stengel 1945). Although recent studies have reported a relatively high incidence (15%) of OC symptoms in schizophrenia (Zaharovits 1990), current literature supports Sir Aubrey Lewis's observation in 1935 that only a small percentage of OCD patients develop schizophrenia. In this chapter we review the clinical and treatment characteristics of schizophrenic patients with OC symptoms with an emphasis on features that distinguish these patients from OCD patients with psychotic features.

Phenomenology

According to the DSM-III-R (American Psychiatric Association 1987), the obsessions or compulsions in OCD must be a significant source of stress to the individual or interfere with social or role functioning. The DSM-III-R criteria also require that the patient show, at least initially, resistance to and insight into the nature of the obsessions and compulsions. As Insel (1984) stated, it is the insight and resistance concerning the internal origin of an obsession that differentiates it from a delusion that is believed to be external and not resisted. This observation highlights the potential difficulty of reliably diagnosing obsessions and compulsions in schizophrenic patients. Fenton and McGlashan (1986), in a retrospective chart review of schizophrenic patients with OC symptoms, reported difficulty with the application of DSM-III-R definitions for obsessions and compulsions, particularly regarding insight and resistance to these symptoms. These authors therefore chose to describe and classify the symptoms behaviorally. Zohar et al. (J. Zohar, Z. Kaplan, J. Benjamin, unpublished manuscript, 1991), reporting on a small series of schizophrenic patients with OC symptomatology, found that with the aid of patient and focused questioning, the subjects investigated were able to distinguish obsessions and compulsions from psychoses. The psychotic symptoms were perceived as ego-syntonic and not resisted, whereas the OC symptomatology was perceived as being ego-dystonic, with varying degrees of resistance reported.

Case Examples

The following case reports of subjects in the study illustrate OC symptomatology in schizophrenic patients in whom both insight and resistance to the symptoms are present.

Case 1

Mr. A., a 27-year-old single male, had a 7-year history of undifferentiated schizophrenia characterized by social isolation, flat affect, impairment in personal hygiene, vagueness, and lack of initiative. During his latest hospitalization, compulsive hand washing and counting of floor tiles, succeeded on each occasion by a stereotyped prayer, were noted. On questioning, he revealed a concern that he had tread on God on one of the tiles and must identify the particular tile involved in order to undo the sacrilege. Although Mr. A. had insight into the complete irrationality of these thoughts, attempts to avoid the ritualistic behavior caused him incapacitating anxiety. Hence, the preoccupation and its associated behavior were therefore interpreted as obsessions and compulsions, respectively.

Case 2

Mr. B., a 23-year-old single male, had a 4-year history of schizophrenia, schizoaffective type, with multiple hospitalizations because of paranoid delusions accompanied by depressive or elated affect. During these psychotic exacerbations he would often lock himself in his room for fear he might otherwise act out aggressive impulses toward his father. Unlike the paranoid delusions, which were ego-syntonic, the aggressive impulses were stereotyped, intrusive, and ego-dystonic, and therefore were interpreted as obsessional in nature.

Case 3

Ms. C., a 30-year-old single female with schizophrenia, schizoaffective type, had had 12 lengthy admissions in the last 7 years because of psychotic episodes characterized by psychomotor agitation, promiscuous sexual behavior, auditory hallucinations, and preoccupation with religious themes. She had never achieved a full remission between exacerbations. During her last hospitalization she complained once more of persistent religious preoccupations. She was quite devoid of insight, yet in order to combat these religious preoccupations she began to count tiles, walk backward, and bite her finger, behavior that was interpreted as a compulsion.

Case 4

Mr. D., an 18-year-old single male, was diagnosed as schizophrenic since the onset of delusions of thought broadcasting and persecution, together with an intellectual and social decline, at the age of 14. In addition, he was preoccupied with the subject of numbers. He asked family members the same questions about numbers over and over again. If prevented from doing so, he became agitated to the point of violence. During past (but not present) admissions this behavior was accompanied by repetitive hand washing. Mr. D. was well aware that his repeated questions were senseless and offensive, but he was powerless to control his behavior. Consequently, the questions were interpreted as a compulsion, while the preoccupation with numbers was interpreted as an obsession.

Case 5

Mr. E., a 36-year-old divorced male, suffered from hebephrenic schizophrenia for 20 years and had been an inpatient for 11 years. Neuroleptics and ECT had no significant effect. For many years he had been preoccupied with the cleanliness of his clothing, an issue that caused him great distress, as well as the question of who created him. He would repeat the phrase "It's nothing" or "It's only in my head" over and over, and then insist that the staff say the same thing to him. Afterward, he disowned this behavior and apologized profusely. This repetition and insistence that the staff copy him was interpreted as compulsive in nature.

Comorbidity

The comorbidity of patients with schizophrenia and OC symptomatology has not been well documented. In one study, Fenton and McGlashan (1986) reported that schizophrenic patients with OC symptoms demonstrated a poorer long-term outcome than schizophrenic patients without OC symptoms. The authors discussed three hypotheses regarding this finding. The first is that schizophrenia with OC symptomatology represents a rare but "virulent" subtype of schizophrenia. The second explanation takes into consideration the possibility that these patients suffer simultaneously from two separate disorders, and, therefore, their poorer outcome may reflect the cumulative or multiplicative effect of these two disorders. The third hypothesis suggests that the prognostic significance of OC symptoms may derive primarily from their chronic nature.

Although these issues require further investigation, it seems quite clear that persistent OC symptoms do appear to be a powerful predictor of outcome.

Differential Diagnoses

Obsessive-Compulsive Disorder With Psychotic Features

According to the DSM-III-R, the senseless character of the obsessions or compulsions is an essential diagnostic criterion for OCD. During the course of the illness, however, the patient at times may lose insight into the senselessness of the obsession. Insel and Akiskal (1986) reviewed case reports of OCD patients with psychotic features and found that the loss of insight into obsessions was related to the onset of psychotic features in these patients. Although the frequency of psychosis in OCD remains unclear, Lelliott et al. (1988) reported that one-third of the 49 OCD patients in their study perceived their obsessions as rational.

This shift from a "senseless" irrational obsession to a "senseful" and rational obsession may also be accompanied by changes in the ego-dystonic quality of the obsession. An example of such a transformation is presented by Insel and Akiskal (1986), who described a case report of a 25-year-old man hospitalized because of compulsive checking of many years duration. At the time of admission the patient expressed a fear that he had inadvertently poisoned children's juice at his place of work. He perceived these thoughts as both embarrassing and irrational. Over the course of his hospitalization there was a deterioration in his status, with a marked change occurring in the quality of his obsession. Although the content remained unchanged, the "obsession" took on delusional properties. He came to believe that various authorities were convinced of his guilt and that he would be punished for crimes he had not committed.

Lelliott et al. (1988) described the case of a 22-year-old soldier who believed that his rituals prevented wars from happening. When he was seen at the time of the battle for the Falkland Islands, he was spending many hours in ritualistic counting and checking so that conflict would not escalate. He was convinced that his fears were justified and felt that others were mistaken in not sharing them. He could not, however, explain how his actions could affect global events. This case, too, illustrates how an obsession may attain delusional proportions.

At times the shift from obsession to delusion is not abrupt or distinct, but fluctuates between the two. Robinson et al. (1975) described the case of a young woman with repeated hospital admissions because of "obsessive psychosis." In one of her admissions she was obsessed with the thought that she had killed somebody in the department where she worked. She was unable to give any clear details surrounding this obsession. Although she reported at times that the idea appeared to her bizarre and unreal, at other times she would spend time searching the department in an effort to find out who was missing so that she could remember whom she had killed.

Robinson et al. (1975), in their follow-up of 36 cases of "obsessive psychosis," observed that these patients differed from schizophrenic patients in several domains. The emotional life of patients suffering from obsessive psychosis was not shallow, and there did not appear to be any intellectual impairment, even in chronic cases. Neither loosening of association nor any hallucinations were observed. This latter finding differs from that reported by Rasmussen and Tsuang (1986), who found that 2 of the 44 OCD patients in their study manifested hallucinations.

These cases challenge the DSM-III-R criteria for senselessness of the obsession and support Lewis's (1935) view that "the recognition that the obsession is senseless is not an essential characteristic of an obsession" (p. 325) and that "critical appraisal of the obsession and recognition that it is absurd is not always present" (p. 326).

Schizotypal Personality Disorder With Concomitant Obsessive-Compulsive Disorder

Jenike et al. (1986) described a subgroup of OCD patients who were refractory to the usual therapeutic regimens. These nonresponders were characterized by the presence of odd speech, ideas of reference, occasional paranoia, and frequent evidence of magical thinking. Depersonalization and derealization were also common. Most of these patients fulfilled the criteria for schizotypal personality disorder. The authors referred to these patients as "schizo-obsessive." These patients did not manifest psychotic symptoms characteristic of schizophrenia. The authors reported that the presence of this personality disorder predicted a poor response to pharmacotherapy and behavior therapy. They recommended that more effective management of these patients could be achieved by treating primarily the personality disorder with supportive therapy, limit setting, family therapy, and patient involvement in structured living situations and treatment programs.

Epidemiology

Early investigators (Jahrreiss 1926; Rosen 1957) described OC symptoms in between 1% and 3.5% of schizophrenic patients. However, in a recent survey (Zaharovits 1990) the presence of OC symptoms in schizophrenia reached 15%. This increase in the percentage of schizophrenic patients with OC symptoms may parallel recent reports of the increased prevalence of OCD in the general population (Robins et al. 1984).

One possible explanation for this increase in the prevalence of OCD may lie in growing medical awareness regarding this disorder. Although it is possible that there has been an increase in the prevalence of this disorder, this seems unlikely. If the high percentage of schizophrenic patients with OC symptoms is confirmed in other studies, it again raises the possibility of a common pathogenesis of these two disorders.

Dopamine and Obsessive-Compulsive Symptomatology

Numerous studies have provided several lines of evidence supporting the hypothesis that dopaminergic dysfunction plays a central role in schizophrenia. In a recent report Goodman et al. (1990) proposed that some forms of OCD may also involve a dysfunction in the dopaminergic as well as serotonergic systems. The authors reviewed preclinical and clinical data supporting this conclusion. The following are some of the more salient findings:

1. High doses of amphetamines (Creese and Iversen 1974; Wallach 1974), which increase dopamine transmission, as well as other dopaminergic agents such as bromocriptine, apomorphine, and L-dopa, have been shown to induce stereotypies in animal models (Creese and Iversen 1974; Loew et al. 1980 Wallach 1974; Wallach and Gershon 1970).

2. In rats, acute administration of the D_2 agonist quinpirole induced perseveration of routes (i.e., sequence of paths taken in open field) in animal studies (Eilam et al. 1989).

3. Several studies have reported stimulant-induced behaviors in humans that resemble naturally occurring OC symptoms (Koizumi 1985; Randrup and Munkvad 1967).

4. There is a high prevalence of OC symptoms in postencephalitic parkinsonian patients, the neuropathology of which involves the basal ganglia and dopamine-containing cells of the ventral tegmental area (Devinsky 1983). There are also reports by Sacks (1983) that the OC symptoms in these patients were exacerbated by L-dopa treatment.

These findings suggest a possible role for dopaminergic hyperfunctioning in the pathophysiology of OC symptoms. However, another study (Insel et al. 1983) demonstrated that single doses of D-amphetamine were actually associated with improvement in severity of OCD. In their review, Goodman et al. (1990) reported that combining neuroleptic treatment and ongoing therapy with selective serotonin reuptake blockers may reduce the severity of OC symptoms in those patients who do not respond to the serotonin reuptake blockers alone. The possible role of the brain dopaminergic system in the pathophysiology of both OCD and schizophrenia is fascinating. However, a full discussion of the possible roles of dopamine, serotonin, and dopamine-serotonin interactions in these disorders is outside the scope of this chapter.

Treatment

Traditional clinical wisdom emphasizes the potential of monoamine reuptake blockers to exacerbate schizophrenic psychosis (Siris et al.

1987). Three double-blind, placebo-controlled studies that examined the use of combined neuroleptic-antidepressant therapy in anergic depressed schizophrenic patients and in actively psychotic schizophrenic patients (Dufresne et al. 1988; Kramer et al. 1989; Siris et al. 1987) suggest that the combination did not cause the patients to become more psychotic. However, use of this therapy may have increased the risk of slower or incomplete resolution of the psychosis (Kramer et al. 1989).

Studies have demonstrated that serotonergic drugs like clomipramine are effective in the treatment of OCD (Zohar and Insel 1988). Based on these findings, Zohar et al. (J. Zohar, Z. Kaplan, J. Benjamin, unpublished manuscript, 1991) designed an open pilot study aimed at exploring the possible benefit of adding "anti-obsessive" medication to the antipsychotic regimen of schizophrenic inpatients.

Five schizophrenic patients, aged 18 to 38, entered the study. The patients were selected on the basis of past and current histories of persistent, intrusive thoughts that they recognized as originating within themselves and that, at least part of the time, they attempted to suppress or ignore. In all cases where compulsions were present, they were repetitive, goal-oriented behaviors designed to neutralize or prevent the discomfort associated with the obsessions. All five patients had a substantial reduction of previously persistent OC symptoms 3 to 6 weeks after the addition of clomipramine, 250 to 300 mg/day, to their ongoing antipsychotic treatment. In four of the five cases this improvement in OC symptomatology was associated with a parallel improvement in psychotic behavior, and only in one case was the addition of clomipramine followed by an exacerbation of psychotic symptoms. With cessation of the clomipramine treatment, all five patients demonstrated a relapse of their OC symptoms within 2 to 4 weeks. In two cases clomipramine was not reinstituted: one patient declined to return to care, and in another patient, whose psychosis appeared to have been aggravated by clomipramine, a second attempt seemed inadvisable. In the remaining three cases a second course of clomipramine was associated once again with improvement in OC symptoms.

A limitation of this report, as indeed of any case report, is the potential overrepresentation of positive results. Because we are not aware of previous attempts to treat OC symptoms in schizophrenic patients with clomipramine, we cannot speculate on the frequency of negative results, if these have in fact occurred but gone unreported. However, all of the schizophrenic patients with OC symptoms offered clomipramine treatment were included in this study.

The approach employed by the authors in this study was to combine specific treatment (clomipramine) for particular symptoms (obsessions and/or compulsions) with appropriate treatment (neuroleptics) for the "principal" diagnosis (schizophrenia). This approach, which was found to be fruitful in this open pilot study, lends support to the concept of symptomatic as opposed to "syndromic" treatment in psychiatry (van Praag et al. 1990). Based on this concept we suggest that the treatment of OCD with psychotic features should consist of a combination of "antiobsessional" drugs and "antipsychotic" treatment.

Conclusions

In this chapter we described two groups of patients that may manifest obsessive-compulsive and psychotic symptoms concurrently. These two groups differ greatly from each other with regard to prognosis. Patients suffering from OCD with psychotic decompensation represent a small percentage of severely ill OCD patients.

The very high prevalence (15%) of OC symptoms in schizophrenic patients, if confirmed in additional studies, may indicate a subtype of schizophrenia. The identification of such a subtype may have clinical importance, as such patients may show preferential response to pharmacotherapy. Furthermore, it may be hypothesized that this subtype of schizophrenia could benefit from atypical neuroleptics (e.g., clozapine) that have serotonergic properties.

References

American Psychiatric Association: Diagnostic and Statistical Manual of Mental Disorders, 3rd Edition, Revised. Washington, DC, American Psychiatric Association, 1987

Creese I, Iversen SD: The role of forebrain dopamine systems in amphetamine-induced stereotyped behavior in the rat. Psychopharmacologia 39:345–357, 1974

Devinsky O: Neuroanatomy of Gilles de la Tourette's syndrome: possible midbrain involvement. Arch Neurol 40:508–514, 1983

Dufresne RL, Kass DJ, Becker RE: Bupropion and thiothixene versus placebo and thiothixene in the treatment of depression in schizophrenia. Drug Development Research 12:259–266, 1988

Eilam D, Golani I, Szechtman H: D2-agonist quinpirole induces perseveration of routes and hyperactivity but no perseveration of movement. Brain Res 490:255–257, 1989

Fenton WS, McGlashan TH: The prognostic significance of obsessive-compulsive symptoms in schizophrenia. Am J Psychiatry 143:437–441, 1986

Goodman WK, McDougle CJ, Price LH, et al: Beyond the serotonin hypothesis: a role for dopamine in some forms of obsessive-compulsive disorder? J Clin Psychiatry 51 (no 8, suppl):36–43, 1990

Insel TR (ed): New Findings in Obsessive-Compulsive Disorder. Washington, DC, American Psychiatric Press, 1984, p 10

Insel TR, Akiskal HS: Obsessive-compulsive disorder with psychotic features: a phenomenologic analysis. Am J Psychiatry 143:1527–1533, 1986

Insel TR, Hamilton JA, Guttmacher LB: D-Amphetamine in obsessive-compulsive disorder. Psychopharmacology (Berlin) 8:231–235, 1983

Jahrreiss W: Über Zwangsvorstellungen im Verlauf der Schizophrenie. Archiv für Psychiatrie 77:740–788, 1926

Jenike MA, Baer L, Minichiello WE, et al: Concomitant obsessive-compulsive disorder and schizotypal personality disorder. Am J Psychiatry 143:530–532, 1986

Koizumi HM: Obsessive-compulsive symptoms following stimulants (letter). Biol Psychiatry 20:1332–1333, 1985

Kramer MS, Voegl WH, DiJohnson C, et al: Antidepressants in "depressed" schizophrenic inpatients. Arch Gen Psychiatry 46:922–928, 1989

Lelliott PT, Noshirvani HF, Basoglu M, et al: Obsessive-compulsive beliefs and treatment outcome. Psychol Med 18:697–702, 1988

Lewis A: Problems of obsessional illness. Proc R Soc Med 29:324–336, 1935

Loew DM, Vigouret JM, Jaton A: Neuropharmacology of bromocriptine and dihydroengotoxine, in Ergot Compounds and Brain Function: Neuroendocrine and Neuropsychiatric Aspects. Edited by Goldstein M. New York, NY, Raven, 1980, pp 63–74

Randrup A, Munkvad HM: Stereotyped activities produced by amphetamine in several animal species and man. Psychopharmacologia 11:300–310, 1967

Rasmussen SA, Tsuang MT: Clinical characteristics and family history in DSM-III obsessive-compulsive disorder. Am J Psychiatry 143:317–322, 1986

Robins LN, Helzer JE, Weissman MM: Lifetime prevalence of specific psychiatric disorders in three sites. Arch Gen Psychiatry 41:949–958, 1984

Robinson H, Winnik A, Weiss A: "Obsessive psychosis": justification for a separate clinical entity. Israel Annals of Psychiatry and Related Disciplines 13:137–141, 1975

Rosen I: The clinical significance of obsessions in schizophrenia. Journal of Mental Science 103:778–785, 1957

Sacks O: Awakenings. New York, Dutton, 1983

Siris SG, Morgan V, Fagerstrom R, et al: Adjunctive imipramine in the treatment of postpsychotic depression: a controlled trial. Arch Gen Psychiatry 44:533–539, 1987

Stengel E: A study of some clinical aspects of the relationship between obsessional neurosis and psychotic reaction types. Journal of Mental Science 41:166–187, 1945

van Praag HM, Asnis GM, Kahn RS, et al: Monoamines and abnormal behaviour: a multi-aminergic perspective. Br J Psychiatry 157:723–734, 1990

Wallach MB: Drug-induced stereotyped behavior: similarities and differences, in Neuropsychopharmacology of Monoamines and Their Regulatory Enzymes. Edited by Usdin E. New York, Raven, 1974, pp 241–260

Wallach MB, Gershon S: A neuropsychopharmacological comparison of D-amphetamine, L-dopa and cocain. Neuropharmacology 5:135–142, 1970

Zaharovits I: Obsessive compulsive symptoms in schizophrenia, in New Research Program and Abstracts, 143rd annual meeting of the American Psychiatric Association, New York, May 1990, NR139, p 99

Zohar J, Insel TR: Diagnosis and treatment of obsessive-compulsive disorder. Psychiatric Annals 18:168–171, 1988

Chapter 11

Cognitive-Behavioral Approaches to Obsessive-Compulsive–Related Disorders

Stephen C. Josephson, Ph.D.
Elizabeth Brondolo, Ph.D.

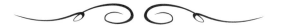

A number of different psychiatric conditions have been associated with obsessive-compulsive disorder (OCD). Some of these disorders, including body dysmorphic disorder, hypochondriasis, and pathological jealousy, have obsessive ruminations and avoidant behavior as primary characteristics. Other disorders, including pathological gambling and compulsive sexual activity, Tourette's syndrome, and trichotillomania, have repetitive and compulsive behaviors as the primary complaint.

These obsessive-compulsive–related disorders (OCRDs) have been treated with a variety of behavioral interventions, some of which have been modeled after approaches used for treating classic OCD symptoms (e.g., hand washing or checking). There are few empirical studies evaluating the treatment of OCRDs. Instead the literature consists largely of uncontrolled case studies, with a few exceptions (Azrin 1990; Azrin et al. 1980a, 1980b; McConaghy et al. 1983). In this chapter, behavioral interventions for the OCRDs listed above will be reviewed, and issues in clinical management and research methodology will be raised. Special attention is focused on the implications of treatment outcome for an understanding of the relation between these disorders and OCD.

Treatment of Obsessive-Compulsive Disorder

Obsessive-compulsive disorder has been conceptualized as an anxiety disorder, and the methods used effectively for anxiety disorders such as social phobia, agoraphobia, and panic disorder have been applied to the treatment of OCD as well. Treatment for OCD involves multiple interventions, targeting the obsessive thoughts, anxious and depressed feelings, and compulsive actions associated with the disorder. In the first stage of treatment, patients may be asked to self-monitor by, for example, keeping diaries that provide detailed descriptions of ritualistic behaviors and intrusive thoughts. Methods for enhancing motivation (e.g., spouse training) may be provided. Relaxation training may be offered to help patients reduce distress during anxiety-producing situations. Coping self-talk that uses humor or anger against the fear may be included (e.g., "I refuse to wash my hands even if they fall off").

Reassurance (i.e., telling patients that their fears are unfounded) is avoided. Reassurance does not provide an effective long-term reduction in obsessional fears and seems to be the functional equivalent of a compulsive ritual. Patients' anxiety levels temporarily decrease when reassurance is given, but rise again soon after the support is removed.

The second level of treatment generally involves exposure and response prevention methods. Response prevention means stopping the patient from engaging in the compulsive behavior (e.g., preventing him or her from washing hands). A delay or change in the ritual (e.g., a shorter shower) may be a valuable first step to expose the patient to anxiety-evoking situations.

After the construction of a hierarchy of anxiety-provoking triggers, a single manageable situation may be identified. With modeling and prompting, the patient is helped to do something that triggers an obsession or compulsion and then is not permitted to engage in the ritual (e.g., instructed to think about death but prevented from knocking on wood or washing hands). The best outcome seems to occur when the exposure is prolonged and the patient can actually experience a significant rise and then fall in distress during the sessions and when home practice is conducted (Foa et al. 1985).

There is controversy about the mechanisms that contribute to the effectiveness of these interventions (Wilson 1990). Exposure and response prevention may be effective because patients learn new, appropriate behaviors to exhibit in response to anxiety-generating situations. The patients may also habituate to previously arousing cues. Alternatively, treatment may change the way patients think about themselves. As patients learn they can tolerate anxiety-producing situations, they may increase their self-efficacy and believe they can, and should, use noncompulsive means of handling stress. Patients may also learn that certain events are not associated with catastrophic outcomes. Evidence exists to support the primacy of both cognitions and behaviors in determining treatment outcome (Franks 1987).

Across reviewed studies, between 60% and 90% of OCD patients benefit from behavioral treatments that include exposure and response prevention. These patients display reductions in symptoms of between 50% and 80%. However, most treatment outcome studies reflect the effects of treatment when only motivated subjects are included. The actual number of OCD patients who would benefit from current behavioral interventions is likely to be somewhat lower (Griest 1990).

In the following sections, treatments for OCRDs are reviewed. Descriptions of the techniques employed are given in Table 11–1, and information on the reported efficacy of the treatments is presented in Table 11–2.

Cognitive Disorders

Body Dysmorphic Disorder

"Dysmorphophobia," or body dysmorphic disorder (BDD) as it is now classified by DSM-III-R (American Psychiatric Association 1987), was a term first coined in 1886 by Morselli to refer to a "subjective feeling of ugliness or physical defect which the patient feels is noticeable by others, although his appearance is within normal limits." Behavioral approaches to treating BDD reflect a conception of BDD as an anxiety disorder. Specifically, patients with BDD are extraordinarily distressed over their appearance and are obsessed with, and possibly deluded by, what they experience as a horribly ugly flaw. For example, in one study, patients believed they were overly hairy, were smelly, or had abnormally large facial features (Marks and Mishan 1988).

Acute emotional reactions are triggered by exposure to certain situations (e.g., mirrors, social situations, conversational remarks) and often are followed by avoidance behavior. Patients may show symptoms of depression and have difficulty going out or even answering the doorbell (Marks and Mishan 1988). Checking rituals (e.g., repeated examinations in mirrors, palpation, asking for reassurance) are often present and temporarily reduce distress. Desperate visits to

Table 11–1. Behavior therapy approaches to the treatment of obsessive-compulsive–related disorders

Behavioral techniques	Description
Relaxation	Varied methods generally involving instruction in calm breathing, positive imagery, release of muscle tension, and suggestions of pleasant sensations
Imaginal desensitization	Having patient imagine distressing scenes of increasing intensity while in a state of deep relaxation
In vivo exposure (flooding, saturation, implosion)	Instructing patient to confront anxiety-provoking situations
Response prevention	Inhibition of compulsive ritual (overt and covert), sometimes with assistance
Self-monitoring	Symptom diary to increase awareness of antecedents and consequences (e.g., sexually compulsive patients record urges, number of partners, etc.)
Contingency management	Program of explicit rewards and punishments (tangible or social) for desired negative behaviors (e.g., no hair pulling at home earns new dress)
Social skills training	Training in social behaviors through modeling, rehearsal, and feedback
Thought stopping	Use of subvocalization ("Stop!") to interrupt negative thought sequences
Massed negative practice	Repeated performance of behavior until satiation (e.g., voluntary emission of tic)
Habit reversal[a]	13-step program (see section on Tourette's syndrome)

[a]Components of habit reversal include, among others, self-monitoring, identification of antecedents of behavior, relaxation, competing response training, and evaluation of costs and benefits of treatment.

Table 11–2.   Efficacy of behavior therapy treatments of obsessive-compulsive–related disorders

	BDD	Hyp	Jeal	Sexual comp	Gambl	TS	Trich
Contingency management							
Contracting				P	P	H	P
Controlled engagement				P	P		
Positive reinforcement					P		
Time out					P		
Social skills training							
Communication skills							
Assertiveness			P	P			
Marital therapy			P	P	P		
Social skills	P				P	P	
Habit-reversal program						H	H
Relaxation							
Hypnosis	P						P
Meditation						P	P
Progressive relaxation					P		
Exposure methods							
Systematic desensitization							
Imaginal	H				H		
In vivo		P					
Indirect		P					
Exposure							
Graded in vivo exposure	P	P					
Imaginal exposure	P	P		P			
Maximal flooding							
Implosion							
Paradoxical intervention	P	P		P			
Satiation		P					
Massed negative practice						M	M
Blocking methods							
Thought stopping		H	H, P				
Response prevention	P	P	P	P			
Aversive conditioning							
Covert sensitization			P		M	M	M
Distraction							
Other							
Stimulus control					P		
Self-monitoring		P	P	P		H	P

Note. BDD = body dysmorphic disorder; Hyp = hypochondriasis; Jeal = jealousy; Sexual comp = sexual compulsions; Gambl = gambling; TS = Tourette's syndrome; Trich = trichotillomania. H = helpful by itself; M = mixed results; P = helpful as part of multifaceted treatment. Blanks signify absence of empirical data.

plastic surgeons function as extreme escape solutions to the distress that patients experience.

The few published reports of successful behavioral treatments of BDD are uncontrolled case studies. These studies describe two models of treatment: *systematic desensitization* and *exposure and response prevention*. The treatment programs vary in their choice of dependent measures but generally focus on changing distorted cognitions, anxious feelings, and social avoidance.

Systematic desensitization has been successfully employed with this disorder (Munjack 1978). In this procedure, the patients were asked to develop hierarchies of concerns. For example, in the case of a patient with hypersensitivity about a ruddy complexion, items included "having someone say that your face matches your shirt" and "making a toast with everyone looking." Patients were asked to imagine anxiety-evoking scenes (starting with the least distressing) while remaining relaxed through the use of progressive muscular relaxation. This method incorporates elements of imaginal exposure and the provision of an incompatible response (relaxation) to facilitate counter-conditioning. Following treatment, significant improvements were observed in interpersonal relations; on self- reported measures of anxiety, depression, and obsessional thinking; and on psychological scales.

An in vivo exposure and response prevention program has also been employed to treat BDD in patients with extensive avoidance and checking behaviors (Marks and Mishan 1988). During in vivo exposure sessions, patients were asked, for example, to go to pubs without trying to hide parts of their body, or to check their appearance only once before going out. Adjunctive methods, including social skills training and communication skills training, were also included, and four of five patients studied showed a marked decrease in social anxiety and avoidance.

In sum, from the data available, both systematic desensitization and exposure and response prevention produced increases in social interaction and decreases in avoidance, reassurance seeking, and subjective distress. Some modification in the intensity of disturbed beliefs was reported in several case studies, but the obsessional or delusional ideas about bodily distortions appear to be markedly persistent (Marks and Mishan 1988). The use of antipsychotic or other medications may be required in patients with persistent delusions or depression during behavior therapy.

Hypochondriasis

Hypochondriasis involves an irrational fear of having a disease or the belief that one has a serious disease. Hypochondriacal persons tend to be generally anxious and depressed, scan their bodies vigilantly for symptoms of possible illness, and ruminate about the consequences of these sensations. It is common for individuals with hypochondriasis to believe that they are actually ill and to actively seek reassurance by consulting physicians or reading compulsively about health. Checking behaviors, such as frequent pulse taking, are often also present, as are thoughts about physical vulnerability and catastrophe (e.g., cancer). Phobic avoidance is also common (e.g., exercise, eating "taboo" foods). However, unlike panic disorder patients, who think their palpitations reflect an immediate cardiac crisis, hypochondriacal patients focus on the longer-term, yet life-threatening, significance of their symptoms.

Given the key behavioral aspects of hypochrondriasis, it is curious that there are few treatment evaluations. Kellner (1985) cites efforts to use systematic desensitization, implosion, hypnosis, and thought stopping to treat hypochondriasis, and concludes that these methods hold great promise but need further study. The behavioral programs described below include multiple dependent measures but generally focus on changing phobic thoughts, anxious feelings, and compulsive reassurance seeking.

Thought stopping has been used to treat "phobias of internal stimuli" (Kumar and Wilkinson 1971). Patients were instructed to block intrusive thoughts regarding illness by covertly shouting "STOP!" to themselves and then distracting themselves with pleasant imagery. Therapists modeled and rehearsed the techniques with patients and taught relaxation to reduce generalized anxiety symptoms. The 4-week treatment resulted in a significant reduction in the frequency of phobic thoughts, and all four patients studied remained symptom-free at a 12-month follow-up.

Multifaceted exposure-based interventions have also been used to reduce health preoccupations corresponding to a cyclical model of symptom awareness and reassurance seeking (Salkovskis and Warwick 1986). Salkovskis and Warwick (1986) suggest that as patients think about or experience symptoms, their anxiety levels rise, and the patients then begin seeking reassurance from others. Reassurance is followed by an immediate, but temporary, decrease in anxiety. The anxiety returns later, however, and the cycle of reassurance seeking is repeated. Anxious thoughts are maintained through the negative reinforcement of the reassurance and avoidance behavior. In an 8-week treatment program for hospitalized patients, staff were instructed to avoid providing reassurance to patients. The investigators also used an interesting cognitive strategy in which they presented evidence to the patient and asked the patient to determine if the findings suggested the symptoms were anxiety-related or a function of medical illness. This process of examining beliefs is similar to Beck's cognitive approach to depression (Beck and Emery 1985) and was undertaken to minimize the overvalued beliefs characteristic of hypochondriasis. Decreases in anxiety and reassurance seeking were observed in the patients examined (Salkovskis and Warwick 1986).

Exposure and response prevention methods were also employed with 17 patients with illness phobias and hypochondriasis (Warwick and Marks 1988). The treatment was more explicitly comparable to standard behavioral treatments for OCD and consisted of in vivo exposure to the feared situation (e.g., hospitals), response prevention (e.g., no reassurance), satiation (e.g., writing down concerns many times), and paradox (e.g., trying to have a heart attack while exercising). Relatives were provided with the opportunity to develop skills in refusing to reassure the patients. A number of different self-report measures of distress and handicap in different settings indicated a significant improvement on measures of both fear and social functioning in over a third of the patients.

Finally, a single case report described the treatment of a man with heart-attack phobia using a "multifaceted exposure program" (Tearnan et al. 1985). The authors utilized in vivo, imaginal, and "indirect" exposure methods as well as progressive muscle relaxation training.

With the imaginal exposure, the patient was asked to imagine a frightening narration and listen to a taped version of it at home until habituation occurred. In vivo procedures included both homework tasks (e.g., exercise, visits to a coronary care unit) and within-session exposure to bogus heart rate feedback and sudden loud noise. The indirect exposure strategies involved watching a videotaped model simulate a heart attack, reading graphic and sometimes fabricated materials on heart disease, and listening to recordings of his children behaving raucously. Results were encouraging, with the patient demonstrating a decline in Valium usage and health care visits, as corroborated by spouse reports of progress.

In summary, exposure and response prevention methods have been key components of multifaceted treatment programs for patients with hypochondriasis. Thought stopping, relaxation, satiation, paradox, and cognitive evaluation have also been employed. Generally, good results for multifaceted program of studies are noted, although the number of available studies is limited. Treatment seems effective in decreasing anxiety, reassurance seeking, and social avoidance.

Pathological Jealousy

Jealousy is a common emotional state that may reach pathological dimensions in individuals with and without coexisting psychiatric disorders. Morbid jealousy may resemble OCD in some patients when they display intrusive, dystonic ruminations and associated checking rituals (e.g., opening mail, checking underwear for stains). While some jealous patients may be delusional in their beliefs, others recognize the irrational nature of their thoughts and vacillate along a continuum of uncertainty and conviction. Alternating cycles of rage and remorse may develop with significant potential for violence and suicide (Docherty and Ellis 1976).

Some case studies have used thought-stopping procedures either in the context of couples communication therapy or as a method of self-regulation of jealous thoughts (Marks 1976; Rosen and Schnapp 1974). Rosen and Schnapp (1974) describe the successful use of thought stopping with a couple who came for help because of an instance of infidelity on the wife's part that left both spouses in extreme distress. The husband experienced uncontrollable jealous ruminations and relentlessly interrogated his wife concerning her extramarital behavior. The wife maintained his behavior by offering reassurance. The authors taught both partners to use thought stopping to break the communication cycle of jealous questions and reassurance. When the husband initiated questioning, the wife was instructed to say "No!" loudly, and the husband was instructed to say "No" covertly. Both patients reported rapid distraction from jealous thoughts and a subsequent ability to control these destructive communications using covert thought stopping.

Thought stopping has also been employed for the self-regulation of morbid jealousy (Marks 1976). In one case study the patient was trained in three sessions to snap an elastic wristband when jealous thoughts occurred. Following several trials with this aversive technique, the patient was able to have the thoughts remit simply by staring at the band and imagining the sting. Gains were maintained at a 3-month follow-up.

A more comprehensive behavioral approach to jealousy has addressed the often related features of low self-esteem, assertive difficulties, and sexual and marital complaints (Cobb and Marks 1979). In this study the treatment package consisted of multiple components, including communication skills training, self-monitoring of jealous thoughts, and in vivo exposure methods. Training in self-regulated exposure and recognition of jealousy-evoking cues was included. In vivo exposure (i.e., exposing the husband to clues believed to indicate infidelity) was found to be too stressful. A form of response prevention (i.e., differential reinforcement) in which the wife answered only nonjealous questions was also included. Results indicate that while jealous behavior decreased substantially, jealous thoughts did not change in intensity or duration.

In sum, case studies provide support for the use of thought stopping, either as part of couples communication therapy or as a self-management technique, to address jealous ruminations. The clinical examples underscore the need for flexible and multifaceted treatment of obsessional jealousy. The depth of rage and the propensity for violent acting out are serious considerations when implementing procedures such as exposure and response prevention, which evoke considerable anxiety. Careful and ongoing assessment of the patient's mental status should accompany applications of these methods.

Compulsive Behavior Disorders

Tourette's Syndrome

Tourette's syndrome (TS) is characterized by multiple repetitive and rapid motor tics and vocal noises that vary in intensity and controllability. Initial behavioral work on TS conceptualized the motor and vocal tics as learned behaviors whose occurrence was a function of specific environmental contingencies or internal reinforcements (self-stimulation or anxiety reduction). A variety of behavior therapy techniques have been implemented in the treatment of tic disorders, as reviewed in more detail elsewhere (Azrin and Peterson 1988). Summaries of the findings are presented below.

Self-monitoring has been reported to be an effective intervention when used either alone or in conjunction with other therapies (Azrin and Peterson 1988; Billings 1978). Self-monitoring includes recording the frequency of tics and vocalizations using paper and pencil or wrist counters. One or more symptoms may be monitored throughout the day or for predetermined periods or situations. Self-monitoring may allow patients to become more aware of the antecedents and consequences of their tics and thus potentially be better able to develop covert procedures for managing symptoms.

More comprehensive and directive contingency management procedures have also been successfully employed. For example, in one successful program, rewards were given when the patient suppressed tics and displayed appropriate social behavior, and withheld when the patient displayed tics or utterances (Doleys and Kurtz 1974). Positive reinforcement may improve the subject's motivation to control tics. Contingency management programs may also be effective because they provide consistent and accurate feedback to the patient. This feedback may otherwise be unavailable, because people interacting with individuals with TS often attempt to ignore the tics.

Punishment procedures (e.g., electric shock, time out, verbal reprimands) have also been employed to treat TS, but these methods have generally produced short-term gains with no long-term maintenance, and their use is generally contraindicated for ethical concerns (Azrin and Peterson 1988).

Relaxation procedures, such as Jacobsonian muscle relaxation and deep breathing, may be useful adjuncts to treating TS because of their anxiety-reducing properties. Studies have not evaluated the use of relaxation training as the sole intervention for TS, and the available data indicate that this type of procedure reduces the frequency of tics during the sessions but has minimal generalization outside the sessions (Azrin and Peterson 1988; Canavan and Powell 1981). Nonetheless, relaxation procedures may have desirable "side effects" and be of benefit to patients seeking to manage periods of high stress more effectively.

In *massed negative practice* procedures, patients practice the tics repetitively and continuously, because this is hypothesized to satiate the patients' need to perform the tics (Storms 1985). The data on the effectiveness of massed negative practice are mixed, and some authors have noted an exacerbation of symptoms following this type of procedure (Hollandsworth and Baisinger 1978). Currently, it remains unclear which patients benefit from mass negative practice.

Habit reversal is a 13-step program developed by Azrin (1973) and others for use with a variety of nervous habits. Steps include, among others, self-monitoring of the frequency and topography of the tics, identification of the antecedents of the behavior, relaxation training, development of social support, and reviews of the costs and benefits of efforts to reduce tic severity. One of the most critical components of the intervention is *competing response training,* in which subjects perform physical actions that are incompatible with engaging in the tic (e.g., maintaining the head in a forward position and tensing neck muscle when the urge to swing the head to the side occurs).

In several case studies, habit reversal has been demonstrated to be effective in reducing the frequency of tics, with results being noticeable to others and the patients' behavior being rated as more socially appropriate (Finney et al. 1983; Franco 1981). In addition, Azrin et al. (1980a) reported on a clinical comparison between massed negative practice and habit reversal in a sample of patients with unspecified tic disorders. The authors found habit reversal to be significantly more effective in reducing tics, with the majority of habit-reversal patients displaying significant improvement after the first day of treatment and maintaining these gains at follow-up. In a more recent empirical evaluation, the effectiveness of habit reversal has been further substantiated (Azrin and Peterson 1990). To some extent, habit-reversal procedures may be viewed as a form of awareness with response prevention—that is, the competing response serves as a form of response prevention.

In summary, a variety of behavioral techniques are available for the treatment of TS, and substantial treatment success has been reported for habit reversal, self-monitoring, and contingency management. Decreases in the urge to engage in a tic as well as in the frequency of tic behavior have been noted (Azrin and Peterson 1988). Given the multiple symptoms often co-occurring with TS, such as attention deficit, social skills deficits, hyperactivity, and obsessive and compulsive behavior, multicomponent treatment programs may produce the best overall outcome. Social skills training, educational remediation, stress management, and medication may all serve as useful adjunctive treatments for patients with TS (Ostfeld 1988).

Trichotillomania

Trichotillomania is characterized by chronic hair pulling involving the face (beard, eyebrows, eyelashes), head, or body. Behavior therapists have described trichotillomania as a learned "nervous habit," often occurring in response to anxiety or boredom, and maintained in part because the behavior is associated with anxiety reduction and self-stimulation. Behavioral treatments include self-monitoring, self-managed contingency contracting, covert sensitization, massed negative practice, and habit reversal, as reviewed in detail elsewhere (Friman et al. 1984). Summaries of the findings are presented below.

Several studies utilize treatment packages comprised of self-monitoring of hair pulling plus contingency management programs—that is, either a reward for inhibiting hair pulling or a negative consequence for the urge to pull or for the actual behavior (Friman et al.

1984). Self-monitoring generally involves having the subject count the incidence of hair pulling, the number of hairs pulled, or the time spent each day in hair pulling. Investigators also encourage patients to be aware of the chain of behaviors (including raising the hand to the face) that precede actual hair pulling (Stevens 1984). Others require daily collection of hair samples to corroborate self-report data and suggest that hair collecting improves the ability of self-monitoring to reduce hair pulling (Bayer 1972). Being confronted with the evidence of one's self-destructive behavior and having to show this "evidence" to the therapist may serve as a sufficiently uncomfortable experience to motivate efforts at self-control.

Other programs have paired self-monitoring with aversive consequences such as saying "No," snapping a rubberband against the wrist, or performing sit-ups following the urge to pull hair or the hair pulling itself (MacNeil and Thomas 1976; Stevens 1984). Covert sensitization procedures, in which subjects imagine highly stressful or aversive thoughts, can also be used to punish hair-pulling urges or behavior (Bornstein and Rychtarik 1978).

Positive reinforcement for inhibiting hair pulling may also be a useful component of treatment (Friman et al. 1984). In the case of young children or severely developmentally delayed persons, contingencies can be imposed by a supervising adult. The treatment outcome can be enhanced through the coordination of treatment efforts at home and school (Nelson 1982). These contingency management procedures have generally been effective in reducing hair pulling, whether the consequences have been self-managed or imposed by others (Friman et al. 1984).

Habit-reversal programs, described in more detail in the section on Tourette's syndrome, have also been employed to treat trichotillomania. In case studies (Rosenbaum and Ayllon 1981; Tarnowski et al. 1987) and in a randomized comparison of habit reversal and massed negative practice (Azrin et al. 1980b), habit reversal has been demonstrated to be an effective treatment for hair pulling. The results of the comparison study are particularly impressive given that subjects only received a single face-to-face treatment session of 2.5 hours in duration. In the Azrin et al. (1980) study, habit reversal produced a 99% improvement in hair pulling after the first day of treatment, and 18 of the 19 members of the habit-reversal group displayed less than one incident of hair pulling at a 4-week follow-up. Decreases in the urge to pull hair were also reported, although these changes need more systematic exploration. These findings contrast with the effects for massed negative practice, which produced about a 60% decrease after one day of treatment, with 7 out of 15 subjects displaying one or fewer incidents per day of hair pulling at the 4-week follow-up.

In addition, a cognitive factor, *client perceptions of self-control,* has been emphasized in at least three studies (Fleming 1984; Hall and McGill 1986; Stevens 1984). Hall and McGill (1986) employed hypnotic suggestion to improve patient perceptions of self-control. Other authors encouraged the patients to repeat positive, control-oriented self-statements. In each of the studies cited above, the emphasis on self-control was identified by the patients as having positive effects on other behaviors in addition to the targeted hair pulling. This type of intervention clearly warrants further study.

In sum, habit reversal appears to be the most successful and systematically evaluated of the behavioral treatments for trichotillomania (Friman et al. 1984). Given the degree to which investigators have articulated the treatment components and the relative brevity of implementation, it may be useful to consider employing the full habit-reversal procedure as a first step in the behavioral treatment for many patients. Teaching patients to maximize self-control and to better use their time and cope with feelings of loneliness and boredom may be important adjunctive treatments (Fleming 1984; Hall and McGill 1986).

Compulsive Sexual Behavior

Sexual compulsivity, sexual addiction, sexual impulsivity, and *hypersexuality* are terms to describe a "preoccupation with and strong desire for sex which the individual feels unable to control" (Barth and Kinder 1987, p. 15). These varied terms reflect the diagnostic controversies in the field, and, to date, no objective criteria for this behavior pattern exist. Treatment reports are again limited to the clinical anecdotal variety. In most programs, treatment goals are directed toward "control" of sexual behavior as opposed to absti-nence. The 12-step programs commonly used often include a mix of cognitive, behavioral, dynamic, and family interventions, but these programs also lack systematic evaluations.

A group therapy program utilizing both self-monitoring of sexual thoughts, feelings, and experiences, and graded behavioral contracts with social reinforcement and support, has also been attempted (Quadland 1985). The program included a "buddy system" to help members prevent or limit inappropriate sexual behavior. A self-report comparison before and after treatment indicated that treated subjects showed a reduction in mean current number of different sexual partners per month from 11.5 to 3.3 at 6 months post-treatment.

Multifaceted treatment programs have been employed in several case studies reporting successful (although not objectively evaluated) outcomes (Schwartz and Brasted 1985; Sprenkle 1987). In one program, communication training and assertiveness were taught in a paradoxical fashion to a patient and his wife. The "addict" was instructed to deliberately have sexual feeling for an intensive block of 30 minutes a day and to "thank God for this 'gift'" (Sprenkle 1987). Schwartz and Brasted (1985) described a multifaceted treatment that included covert sensitization, fantasy satiation, progressive relax-ation, cognitive disputation for the underlying irrational beliefs, and assertiveness/problem solving to enhance appropriate social con-duct. Couples therapy to strengthen the committed primary relation-ship was seen as a final component of this multistage approach.

One of the present authors (S.C.J.) has worked with a number of "sexually compulsive" patients using a similar multifaceted approach. Clinical experience suggests that systematic efforts to expose patients to both internal and external triggers of compulsive behavior may result in habituation to the desire for compulsive sex. Exposure and response prevention methods may be employed by instructing patients to fantasize and/or "cruise" possible partners without engag-ing in any actual contact. Masturbatory satiation and reconditioning techniques, as well as efforts to "deglamorize" the experience with reframing methods (e.g., promiscuity is due to insecurity), may prove to be helpful auxiliary tools. Social skills training to improve patients' ability to maintain intimate relationships may also be desirable.

Pathological Gambling

Pathological gambling is characterized by "a chronic and progressive failure to resist impulses to gamble" (American Psychiatric Association 1987, p. 324), with the gambling behavior producing deleterious consequences, including a loss of work, money, and/or family stability (see Chapter 8, this volume). Individuals may begin gambling for the excitement and monetary rewards, but they continue gambling as a distraction or release from anxiety or depression or to avoid further losses. Further incidences of gambling may be initiated by exposure to gambling-related cues such as the sight of a betting shop or of the racing pages in a newspaper.

Aversive conditioning methods have been employed in an attempt to reduce the reinforcing properties of gambling and to generate an aversive or unpleasant consequence associated with engaging in gambling. One example of these procedures is the pairing of electric shock with gambling-related stimuli (e.g., betting shops). Following treatment, patients are believed to avoid the behavior because of anxiety or distress associated with completing the gambling activity. Some studies using aversive therapy report limited efficacy (McConaghy et al. 1983; Seager 1970), whereas others report better results (Goorney 1968).

Alternatively, imaginal desensitization has also been employed to treat the urge to gamble and the gambling behavior itself (McConaghy et al. 1983). McConaghy et al. (1983) suggest that the initial sight of a gambling trigger (i.e., a racing form or slot machine) may generate a sense of anxiety accompanied by an urge to gamble. Failure to satisfy the urge may be associated with distress. The authors describe the cycle in which patients experience distress when unable to complete the gambling activities as a *completion mechanism,* and they hypothesize that this mechanism is instrumental in the maintenance of gambling behavior.

Imaginal desensitization attempts to reduce the anxiety evoked by failure to respond to gambling urges. Subjects are asked to imagine several scenes in which they would normally be tempted to gamble. They envision themselves not gambling and perform relaxation techniques to reduce the accompanying anxiety. For example, patients perform muscle relaxation exercises while imagining scenes from their gambling experiences (e.g., being in a betting shop, placing a bet). The one controlled comparison between aversion therapy and imaginal desensitization reveals that imaginal desensitization is somewhat superior to exclusively aversive treatment in reducing the urge to gamble and gambling behavior (McConaghy et al. 1983).

Multifaceted treatment programs that include training in 1) resistance toward the urge to bet, 2) avoidance of betting shops, 3) positive contingency management for appropriate behavior, and 4) aversive techniques such as covert sensitization, have been largely unsuccessful (Greenberg and Marks 1982). Some success has been reported in a single case study with a multicomponent treatment that included family contingency contracting, positive reinforcement, and aversive techniques such as massed negative practice, time out, and electric shocks (Cotler 1971). The patient was able to limit gambling after 16 sessions, although relapse necessitated "booster" sessions, leading to good results.

A multifaceted comprehensive program modeled after alcohol treatment programs has also been employed in the treatment of pathological gambling. The program included a 28-day inpatient stay with individual and group treatment and involvement in Gamblers Anonymous. Fifty-six percent of the patients enrolled in this program reported that they were abstinent from gambling 6 months after treatment (Taber et al. 1987).

Several authors have emphasized the need for treatment of the marital relationship in treating pathological gambling (Cotler 1971; Greenberg and Marks 1982). Too few studies are available to allow a comparison between programs that do include spouse involvement and those that do not. Given the pervasive effects of compulsive behavior such as pathological gambling, it may be critical to include multiple treatment components and spouse involvement to achieve significant success.

Training in controlled gambling may also be a viable treatment option (Dickerson and Weeks 1979; Rankin 1982). In these programs, patients are presented with a series of rules for limiting the amount and frequency of wagers. In one example, Rankin (1982) reports that a severe gambler was able to adhere to the rules reducing the frequency and intensity of gambling; the patient reported a decrease in gambling urges once he followed the rules for controlled gambling.

In sum, treatments for gambling have included a variety of methods, such as aversive therapy (counter-conditioning), imaginal desensitization, and other cognitive and behavioral techniques. Overall, the results of psychotherapeutic treatments for compulsive gambling have been less than encouraging. There are conflicting data concerning the efficacy of counter-conditioning techniques and some suggestion that these aversive techniques may be better at reducing gambling behavior than in reducing the urge to gamble. Imaginal desensitization procedures appear to be effective in reducing gambling urges and behaviors and merit further evaluation. A more systematic evaluation of the role of marital therapy in reducing gambling behavior is also warranted.

Conclusions

The growing literature on behavioral treatment of OCRDs both fills a treatment void and supports, with qualification, the usefulness of generalizing from OCD treatment research. Most of these "related" disorders have been heretofore difficult to treat and unresponsive to psychoanalytic and many drug treatments. In many cases, multifaceted behavioral regimens, in concert with specific medications, can provide a potent treatment approach.

Methodological Issues

There are a variety of methodological problems common to treatment outcome research in the areas reviewed. First, the bulk of the studies are single case reports, subject to the methodological problems common to these designs (Kazdin 1984), and with limited generalizability to the larger patient population. The cases selected for publication are likely to include highly motivated subjects and those for whom treatment oucome was successful. Negative findings are probably underrepresented.

Few studies included any control groups, making it difficult to differentiate effects due to maturation, to attention, or to the active components of therapy. In future studies it would be important to include active treatment controls, especially in disorders such as pathological gambling and sexual compulsion, for which the confession and sharing of addictive behavior are often a part of self-help treatment and may in fact be as, or more, important than more structured behavioral interventions. Direct comparison between two active treatments, such as that employed in McConaghy et al.'s (1983) study comparing aversion to imaginal desensitization, may be the most effective and appropriate test of treatment efficacy. The clinical comparison of Azrin et al. (1980a) of the use of habit reversal versus massed negative practice is a good example of the types of treatment outcome studies that need to be performed. In addition, controls for maturation or time may be essential for disorders such as TS that have symptoms that naturally wax and wane over time.

Multiple treatment methods including medication or cognitive and behavioral methods were used in almost every study, making it difficult to identify active components of treatment. As is clear from Table 11–2, multiple names for procedurally similar treatments exist, and often operational definitions are lacking in published reports. Consistent, standardized names for techniques need to be established, and strategies to identify the active ingredient(s) or sequencing of multiple components are crucial. In other studies, psychoactive medications are used as part of treatment, making it difficult to determine the independent effects of behavior therapy (Marks and Mishan 1988).

Diagnostic questions make interpretation of the results difficult. For doubting disorders such as BDD and hypochondriasis, it may be critical to develop methods for identifying the cognitive (delusional versus obsessional), affective, imaginal, and behavioral components. Distinguishing between delusions versus obsessional ideation, although difficult, may have implications for treatment outcome given the tenacity of delusional beliefs. Similarly, it is not clear if treatment programs effective for patients with simple tics will also be effective for patients with TS, although recent research on TS patients suggests that habit reversal is quite effective with selected patients (Azrin and

Peterson 1990). In addition, it may be critical to directly assess subjects' motivation as part of the evaluation program.

There is often only one-dimensional data on treatment outcome. It may be important to obtain indices of change in thoughts (doubts), feelings (urges), and actions (compulsions). Treatments may be effective for some, but not all, aspects of a condition (e.g., ruminations do not change but behavior does).

Severity of associative psychopathology should also be considered when evaluating treatment effectiveness. Literature on BDD suggests that some behavioral treatment programs (e.g., Marks and Mishan 1988) may be effective in reducing symptoms and producing behavior change even in patients with severe psychopathology and serious impairments in daily living. Other investigators have suggested that behavioral treatments for trichotillomania are less effective in patients with significant associated psychopathology (Ames 1985).

Treatment Issues

Most treatment studies begin with some form of self-monitoring to provide a baseline and enhance awareness of the problem. Our clinical experience suggests that diary keeping is more effective and practical with compulsive behavior disorders than it is with doubting disorders. Although covert phenomena can be monitored, it requires extensive effort and may not be either accurate or helpful. Exposure-based interventions are best if prolonged and if the patient is able to experience anxiety during the exposure. However, the patient's anxiety levels and beliefs about tolerating distress are evaluated carefully. The literature indicates that for both jealousy and BDD, in vivo exposure methods may prove highly stressful for the patients (Munjack 1978; Rosen and Schnapp 1974). Careful assessment of mental status is appropriate.

Treatment of behavioral avoidance and reductions in compulsive behavior may necessitate additional skills training. For example, as individuals with BDD engage in previously avoided situations, they may benefit from social skills training, and those persons with sexual compulsions may benefit from marital therapy or training to improve the ability to form intimate relationships.

The studies reviewed in this chapter suggest that different approaches may be effective with cognitively based doubting disorders (e.g., jealousy) and compulsive disorders (e.g., sexual compulsions). Treatment of doubting disorders might begin with thought stopping in a conjoint and individual context (see Rosen and Schnapp 1974). Then a gradual and careful exposure may be undertaken, beginning with, for example, images of scenes of infidelity. Response prevention for jealous behaviors would follow, and then relationship deficits and difficulties would be addressed. Ongoing homework might include assignments to engage in relationship enhancement activities (e.g., go out to dinner or spend 15 minutes talking with your spouse), as well as assignments to perform imaginal exposure to scenes that evoke jealousy.

In the case of treatment of compulsive behaviors (e.g., trichotillomania or TS), treatment begins with increasing the patient's awareness of the targeted behavior through self-monitoring. Stimulus control (i.e., avoidance of high-probability situations such as being alone or under stressful circumstances) and habit-reversal procedures might follow. Extensive homework and in-session practice of competing response training are incorporated. If necessary, contingency management techniques may be applied. Cognitive reinforcement with hypnotic suggestions of control and self-efficacy would be employed if palatable to the patient.

Habituation to anxiety-producing stimuli is an assumption of exposure treatments. Unfortunately, not all symptoms reflect anxiety alone. Depression or other negative affects may be associated with cognitive distortions in BDD and jealousy. Similarly, boredom and loneliness may also elicit hair-pulling behavior. Thus, exposure methods may only be partially helpful and may need to be supplemented with methods for coping with other negative affects.

Despite the above caveats, the available literature on OCRDs generally supports the notion that these disorders are "related"—that is, they share a rather selective and preferential response to exposure and response-prevention treatment methods. This is seen clearly in the cognitive disorders (i.e., BDD, hypochondriasis, jealousy), where response prevention of rituals facilitates exposure and often results in diminished distress. The studies on the behavioral treatment of pathological gambling, TS, trichotillomania, and sexual compulsiveness suggest that treatment with OCD-derived methods is appropriate and that the disorders share some links to OCD.

A final question has to do with whether doubting and compulsive disorders differ in response to selected treatments. One can tentatively conclude that the doubting disorders respond best to programs in which patients are encouraged to participate in previously avoided activities and in which reassurance seeking is prevented. Compulsive behavior disorders seem most affected by treatments aimed at teaching the patient to "do something different" (i.e., perform a competing response, etc.). Treatments aimed at reducing the anxiety associated with the failure to perform the behavior also show promise.

In conclusion, behavioral methods appear to hold promise as a treatment for many OCRDs. A greater clarity in both diagnostic markers and components of treatments is needed to allow a thorough evaluation of these behavioral techniques. The future holds promise as more rigorous methodology is applied to a greater number of intensively studied patients. However, many patients will continue to need concomitant medication and other forms of therapy, including social skills training.

References

American Psychiatric Association: Diagnostic and Statistical Manual of Mental Disorders, 3rd Edition, Revised. Washington, DC, American Psychiatric Association, 1987

Ames S: Trichotillomania: a reaction to Friman, Finney, Christophersen (1984). Behavior Therapy 16:328–329, 1985

Azrin NH, Nunn RG: Habit reversal: a method of eliminating nervous habits and tics. Behav Res Ther 11:619–178, 1973

Azrin NH, Peterson AL: Behavior therapy for Tourette's syndrome and tic disorders, in Tourette's Syndrome and Tic Disorders: Clinical Understanding and Treatment. Edited by Cohen DJ, Bruun RD, Leckman JF. New York, Wiley, 1988, pp 237–253

Azrin NH, Peterson AL: Treatment of Tourettes by habit reversal: awaiting list control. Behavior Therapy 21:305–318, 1990

Azrin NH, Nunn RG, Frantz SE: Habit reversal vs negative practice treatment of nervous tics. Behavior Therapy 11:169–178, 1080a

Azrin NH, Nunn RG, Frantz SE: Treatment of hairpulling—a comparative study of habit reversal and negative practice treatment. J Behav Ther Exp Psychiatry 11:13–20, 1980b

Barth R, Kinder B: The mislabeling of sexual impulsivity. J Sex Marital Ther 13:15–23, 1987

Bayer C: Self-monitoring and mild aversion treatment of trichotillomania. J Behav Ther Exp Psychiatry 3:139–141, 1972

Beck A, Emery G: Anxiety Disorders and Phobias: A Cognitive Perspective. New York, Basic Books, 1985

Billings A: Self-monitoring in the treatment of tics: a single subject analysis. J Behav Ther Exp Psychiatry 9:339–342, 1978

Bornstein PH, Rychtarik RG: Multicomponent behavioral treatment of trichotillomania: a case study. Behav Res Ther 16:217–220, 1978

Canavan, A, Powell GE: The efficacy of several treatments of Gilles de la Tourette's syndrome as assessed in a single case. Behav Res Ther 19:549–556, 1981

Cobb JP, Marks IM: Morbid jealousy featuring as obsessive compulsive neurosis: treatment by behavioural psychotherapy. Br J Psychiatry 134:301–305, 1979

Cotler S: The use of different behavioral techniques in treating a case of compulsive gambling. Behavior Therapy 2:579–584, 1971

Dickerson MG, Weeks D: Controlled gambling as a therapeutic technique for compulsive gamblers. J Behav Ther Exp Psychiatry 10:139–141, 1979

Docherty JP, Ellis J: A new concept and finding in morbid jealousy. Am J Psychiatry 133:679–683, 1976

Doleys D, Kurtz P: A behavioral treatment program for the Gilles de la Tourette syndrome. Psychol Rep 35:43–48, 1974

Finney J, Rapoff MA, Hall CL, et al: Replication and social validation of habit reversal treatment for tics. Behavior Therapy 14:116–126, 1983

Fleming I: Habit reversal treatment for trichotillomania: a case study. Behavioral Psychotherapy 12:73–80, 1984

Foa EB, Steketee GS, Ozarow BJ: Behavior therapy with obsessive-compulsives: from theory to treatment, in Obsessive-Compulsive Disorder: Psychological and Pharmacological Treatment. Edited by Mavissakalian M, Turner SM, Michelson L. New York, Plenum, 1985, pp 49–129

Franco DD: Habit reversal and isometric tensing with motor tics. Dissertation Abstracts International 42:3418B, 1981

Franks CM: Behavior therapy: an overview, in Annual Review of Behavior Therapy: Theory and Practice, Vol 10. Edited by Franks CM, Wilson GT, Kendall PC, et al. New York, Guilford, 1987, pp 1–46

Friman PG, Finney JW, Christophersen ER: Behavioral treatment of trichotillomania: an evaluative review. Behavior Therapy 15:249–265, 1984

Goorney AB: The treatment of a compulsive horse race gambler by aversion therapy. Br J Psychiatry 114:329–333, 1968

Greenberg D, Marks I: Behavioural psychotherapy of uncommon referrals. Br J Psychiatry 141:148–153, 1982

Griest JH: Obsessive-Compulsive Disorder: What It Is and How It's Treated. Madison, WI, PSG Publishing, 1990

Hall JR, McGill JC: Hypnobehavioral treatment of self-destructive behavior: trichotillomania and bulimia in the same patient. Am J Clin Hypn 29:39–46, 1986

Hollandsworth JG, Baisinger L: Unsuccessful use of massed practice in the treatment of Gilles de la Tourette syndrome. Psychol Rep 43:671–677, 1978

Kazdin AE: Statistical analysis for single-case experimental designs, in Single-Case Experimental Designs: Strategies for Studying Behavior Change. Edited by Barlow D, Hersen M. New York, Pergamon, 1984, pp 285–321

Kellner R: Functional somatic symptoms and hypochondriasis: a survey of empirical studies. Arch Gen Psychiatry 42:821–833, 1985

Kumar K, Wilkinson JCM: Thought stopping: a useful treatment in phobias of "internal stimuli." Br J Psychiatry 119:305–307, 1971

MacNeil J, Thomas MR: The treatment of obsessive compulsive hair pulling by behavioral and cognitive contingency manipulation. J Behav Ther Exp Psychiatry 7:391–392, 1976

Marks IM: The current status of behavioral psychotherapy: theory and practice. Am J Psychiatry 133:253–261, 1976

Marks IM, Mishan J: Dysmorphophobic avoidance with disturbed bodily perception: a pilot study of exposure therapy. Br J Psychiatry 152:674–678, 1988

McConaghy N, Armstrong MS, Blaszczynski A, et al: Controlled comparison of aversive therapy and imaginal desensitization in compulsive gambling. Br J Psychiatry 142:366–372, 1983

Morselli E: Sulla dismorfofobia e Sulla tafefa. Boll Accad Med 6:110–119, 1886

Munjack D: Behavioral treatment of dysmorphophobia. J Behav Ther Exp Psychiatry 9:53–56, 1978

Nelson WM: A behavioral treatment of childhood trichotillomania: a case study. Journal of Clinical Child Psychology 11:227–230, 1982

Ostfeld BM: Psychological interventions in Gilles de la Tourette's syndrome. Psychiatric Annals 18:417–420, 1988

Quadland M: Compulsive sexual behavior: definition of a problem and an approach to treatment. J Sex Marital Ther 11:121–132, 1985

Rankin H: Control rather than abstinence as a goal in the treatment of excessive gambling. Behav Res Ther 20:185–187, 1982

Rosen R, Schnapp B: The use of a specific behavioral technique (thought-stopping) in the context of conjoint couples therapy: a case report. Behavior Therapy 5:261–264, 1974

Rosenbaum MS, Ayllon T: The habit reversal technique in treating tricho-tillomania. Behavior Therapy 12:473–481, 1981

Salkovskis PM, Warwick HM: Morbid preoccupations, health anxiety and reassurance: a cognitive-behavioral approach in hypochondriasis. Behav Res Ther 24 597–602, 1986

Schwartz M, Brasted W: Sexual addiction. Medical Aspects of Human Sexuality 19:103–107, 1985

Seager CD: Treatment of compulsive gamblers by electrical aversion. Br J Psychiatry 117:545–553, 1970

Sprenkle D: Treating a sex addict through marital sex therapy. Family Relations 36:11–14, 1987

Stevens M: Behavioral treatment of trichotillomania. Psychol Rep 55:987–990, 1984

Storms L: Massed negative practice as a behavioral treatment for Gilles de la Tourette's syndrome. Am J Psychother 39:277–281, 1985

Taber J, McCormick RA, Russo AM, et al: Follow-up of pathological gamblers after treatment. Am J Psychiatry 144:757–761, 1987

Tarnowski KJ, Rosén LA, McGrath ML, et al: A modified habit reversal procedure in a recalcitrant case of trichotillomania. J Behav Ther Exp Psychiatry 18:157–163, 1987

Tearnan BH, Goetsch V, Adams HE: Modification of disease phobia using a multifaceted exposure program. J Behav Ther Exp Psychiatry 16:57–61, 1985

Warwick HMC, Marks IM: Behavioural treatment of illness phobia and hypochondriasis: a pilot study of 17 cases. Br J Psychiatry 152:239–241, 1988

Wilson GT: Fear reduction methods and the treatment of anxiety disorders, in Review of Behavior Therapy. Edited by Franks CM, Wilson GT, Kendall PC, et al. New York, Guilford, 1990, pp 72–102

Chapter 12

The Spectrum of Obsessive-Compulsive–Related Disorders

Daniel J. Stein, M.B.
Eric Hollander, M.D.

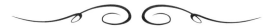

R ecent advances in our understanding of obsessive-compulsive disorder (OCD) have led to increased attention to a number of apparently related disorders. The notion of a spectrum of obsessive-compulsive–related disorders (OCRDs) has gained some popularity (Jenike 1990). In this chapter we review several ways of thinking about the OCD spectrum of disorders. We discuss two traditional clinically based approaches to the OCRDs: that of the early descriptive psychiatrists and that of the classical psychoanalysts. We also note the existence of some less clinically based work on the spectrum of ruminative thoughts. We then consider the relationship between OCD and anxiety, and between OCD and depression. Finally, we consider the evidence of a spectrum between OCD and tic, somatoform, grooming, eating, and impulse disorders. We begin, however, with some comments on the general nature of spectrums of psychopathology and on the value of exploring such spectrums.

Spectrums of Psychopathology

The traditional way of classifying psychiatric disorders entails a categorical approach. Categories are convenient abstractions of clinically important information. They enable the clinician to readily classify different patients, and they may suggest a standard clinical approach.

Categorical classifications may also use hierarchies and groupings to establish relationships between different entities. The various disorders that have been discussed in this book, for example, are classified in DSM-III (American Psychiatric Association 1980) and DSM-III-R (American Psychiatric Association 1987) as quite separate entities that fall in different groupings. Thus, OCD is classified as an anxiety disorder, Tourette's syndrome (TS) as a tic disorder, anorexia nervosa as an eating disorder, body dysmorphic disorder (BDD) and hypochondriasis as somatoform, or perhaps delusional, disorders, trichotillomania as an impulse disorder, and compulsive sexuality as a sexual dysfunction disorder. Because hierarchical considerations apply, the diagnosis of OCD is not given if, for example, the obsessions occur in relation to food and an eating disorder is present. This diagnostic approach provides the clinician with a series of categories that are useful insofar as they allow classification of patients and suggest appropriate clinical approaches. It is also useful, for example, in pointing out that obsessive-compulsive symptoms occur in the context of anorexia nervosa.

On the other hand, there are reasons for employing a dimensional approach in classifying psychopathology. First, the phenomena of the world are only rarely classifiable into categories that are homogeneous, mutually exclusive, and jointly exhaustive. Psychiatric phenomena often fall on a continuum (Kendell 1975). Thus a dimensional approach allows the classification of patients who fall at the border of classical entities or who are otherwise atypical. Similarly, if a patient has the signs and symptoms of two categorical entities, these can be seen as related rather than as merely comorbid. A dimensional perspective may be useful, for example, in working with a patient who appears to fall on the border of OCD and BDD; who simultaneously has TS, trichotillomania, and OCD; or who presents with anorexia nervosa and then goes on to develop OCD.

The DSM manuals note in the introductory section that there are no sharp and natural boundaries that separate mental disorders from normality and from one another. The DSM-III and DSM-III-R emphasize polythetic diagnostic criteria, encourage the use of multiple diagnoses, and include a multiaxial system—all features that make them more flexible than their predecessors, which were more categorical in spirit (Frances 1982). Nevertheless, as can be seen from the classification of OCD and its related disorders, the DSM manuals ultimately retain a focus on *categories* of obsessive-compulsive symptoms. In the remainder of this chapter we will discuss a number of *dimensions* of obsessive and compulsive symptoms.

A second reason for employing a dimensional rather than a categorical approach to psychopathology concerns the different emphasis that each gives to theoretical relationships between disorders. In a categorical system, hierarchies and groupings may be used to suggest relationships between different entities. In a dimensional system, these kinds of relationships may be more overtly specified as particular dimensions are employed to draw attention to particular relationships between different entities. Thus a classification in which rituals and tics fall along a continuous dimension specifies a relationship between OCD and TS. Such a classification may more readily suggest that rituals and tics have a similar etiology, or that they respond to similar treatment.

The introductory section to the DSM manuals argues that these classification systems are atheoretical with respect to the question of etiology. The use of hierarchies and groupings in the manuals does, however, embody some theory about the relationships between disorders. Thus the classification of OCD as an anxiety disorder suggests a relationship between OCD and anxiety. Conversely, the classification of BDD in an entirely different section implies that OCD and BDD are not related. On the other hand, the exclusion criteria in OCD concerning anorexia nervosa point to a relationship between these two disorders. Nevertheless, it may be argued that more detail deserves to be paid to specifying the relationships between different OCRDs. In the remainder of this chapter we will consider possible relationships between the OCRDs at some length.

The categorical and dimensional approaches to psychopathology are not necessarily exclusive. In this book we have already taken a categorical approach to the OCRDs, and we now explore the dimensions along which these disorders fall. It is useful perhaps to list the criteria for considering two categories as dimensionally related. We suggest that diagnostic categories are initially considered along a spectrum if there is considerable symptom overlap. Associated features such as age at onset, clinical course, comorbidity, level of impairment, and prevalence provide further evidence of a spectrum. Similar etiology, as demonstrated by familial linkage, biological markers, or therapeutic (pharmacological) dissection, perhaps provides the most convincing justification for a spectrum.

Obsessive-Compulsive Disorder and Delusions

Early decriptions portray obsessive-compulsive symptoms as related to psychotic states. Westphal contended that obsessions represent a disorder of thinking, and Bleuler regarded obsessive-compulsiveness as a prodrome or variant of schizophrenia (Insel and Akiskal 1986). Both OCD and schizophrenia have early onset, a chronic and debilitating course, and intrusive thoughts and bizarre behavior. OCD patients have been noted to have perceptual distortions (Yaryura-Tobias and Neziroglu 1984). Early authors had limited means with which to investigate organic factors. The etiologic basis for the phenomenological spectrum between OCD and psychosis was, however, considered by these authors to be organic in nature.

Obsessive-compulsive disorder and schizophrenia appear, however, to be readily distinguishable. Although the delusions of schizophrenia can resemble particular obsessional concerns, there is usually less insight into the former. The rituals of schizophrenic patients do not appear to be purposeful and are often in response to what the patient perceives as an external force. Other core positive and negative symptoms of schizophrenia are not present in OCD. Moreover, it has been found that OCD patients only rarely become schizophrenic (Goodwin et al. 1969) and that schizophrenic patients only rarely have OCD (Fenton and McGlashan 1985; Rosen 1957). No family study has suggested a genetic relationship between OCD and schizophrenia, and findings from imaging studies and medication responsivity data do not suggest similarities between the two disorders. In Chapter 10, however, Kindler et al. emphasized the need for further research on schizophrenic patients with obsessive-compulsive symptoms. They pointed out that the prevalence of such symptoms in schizophrenia may be higher than previously thought, that dopamine appears to play a role in both schizophrenia and OCD, and that schizophrenic patients with OCD may respond to serotonin reupake blockers.

Furthermore, there are a considerable number of reports that describe a transition from obsessions to delusions (Insel and Akiskal 1986). The similarity between delusional disorder and OCD has perhaps been underplayed. The two are traditionally distinguished as follows: in OCD, symptoms are recognized as senseless or excessive, while in the delusional disorder, symptoms are, by definition, delusional in intensity. Also, OCD is thought to begin in childhood, adolescence, or early adulthood, while delusional disorder begins in late adulthood. Nevertheless, the obsessional concerns and consequent behaviors of patients with delusional disorder may mimic those of the OCD patient. Conversely, in many cases of OCD, obsessions are ego-syntonic and compulsions are not thought unreasonable (Insel and Akiskal 1986; Stern and Cobb 1978). In both OCD and delusional disorder the obsession or delusion is fairly restricted, and there is no evidence of thought disorder or other positive and negative symptoms.

In addition, the content of such obsessions may be similar in OCD and delusional disorder. Thus a concern with contamination may be present in both. Jealousy may be present in both erotomania and OCD, and somatic concerns may be present in both somatic delusion disorder and OCD. The severe dsyfunction and perhaps poorer prognosis of OCD patients with ego-syntonic symptoms may parallel that seen in psychotic patients. Again, there may be some overlap in treatment response of OCD and delusional disorder (Jenike 1990; McDougle et al. 1990).

Obsessive-Compulsive Disorder and Obsessive-Compulsive Personality Disorder

Freud and subsequent psychoanalysts substituted for the early connection between obsessive-compulsive symptoms and psychosis an emphasis on the concepts of neurosis and character. In his classic volume, Salzman (1968), a contemporary analyst, describes the phenomenology of obsessive-compulsivity as existing on a spectrum between a character problem and a neurotic problem in which symptoms manifest. Both clinical presentations are explicable on the basis of a particular set of underlying dynamic mechanisms, but in the case of the character problem these mechanisms are more functional and more ego-syntonic. In addition, Salzman describes a set of OCD-related disorders, namely phobias and alcoholism. The basis on which he considers these to be related disorders is again the existence of similar underlying psychodynamics. Such disorders as TS, trichotillomania, BDD, hypochondriasis, and anorexia nervosa are not referenced in the book.

Contemporary thinking does not support the notion of OCD as on a spectrum with obsessive-compulsive personality disorder (OCPD). Modern nosology emphasizes the traditional phenomenological distinction between OCD and OCPD patients: the former have ego-dystonic obsessions and compulsions, whereas the latter have ego-syntonic character traits without obsessions and compulsions. However, obsessions and compulsions are sometimes ego-syntonic, and OCPD patients often experience discomfort and disability. Furthermore, some overlap in symptoms may be present—for example, both OCD and OCPD patients may be hoarders, or have extreme moral scrupulosity. Nevertheless, the phenomenological distinction between OCD and OCPD appears statistically reproducible (Pollack 1979). More closely related to the phenomenology of OCD is subclinical OCD—that is, obsessions and compulsions that are only minimally resisted and that do not cause significant distress or dysfunction and therefore do not meet the criteria for OCD (Rachman and Da Silva 1978).

The idea that a particular etiologic mechanism accounts for both

OCD and OCPD has also not received much support. Several studies have indicated that OCPD neither precedes nor is always associated with OCD (Baer et al. 1990; Black 1974; Joffe et al. 1988; Pollack 1987). Conversely, patients with OCPD may not develop other psychiatric disorders, or they may develop psychiatric disorders other than OCD. Neuropsychological studies of patients with OCD (Rosen et al. 1988) and of patients with OCPD (Reed 1977) have not clearly pointed to a continuum between the disorders, although more work needs to be done. Early family studies suggesting increased obsessional traits in relatives of OCD patients, and more recent controlled studies pointing to an increase in OCD in relatives, have been reviewed by Rasmussen and Eisen (1990). These authors argue, however, that further diagnostic clarity between OCD and OCPD is necessary in such work. Finally, although there is a lack of controlled studies, it appears that patients with OCD respond to behavior treatment, while the psychotherapy of choice for OCPD patients is insight oriented.

The relationship between OCD and OCPD nevertheless remains of interest. Swedo et al. (1989b) have suggested that OCPD may develop in some OCD patients as an adaptation to the illness. There are anecdotal reports of OCPD patients experiencing subjective alleviation and improved functioning on serotonergic agents. Understanding the etiologic mechanisms of OCPD may therefore contribute to our knowledge of OCD.

Obsessive-Compulsive Disorder and Rumination

While obsessive-compulsive phenomena have been approached by psychiatrists from a clinical perspective, psychologists have tackled similar phenomena from a somewhat different viewpoint. Martin and Tesser (1989), for example, have explored rumination using a cognitive-psychology framework. They define rumination as conscious thinking directed toward a given object for an extended period of time. The concept therefore refers to a broad range of cognitive phenomena, including problem solving and anticipation as well as a number of different thoughts seen in the clinic, such as negative thoughts in depressed patients and intrusive thoughts in OCD.

Martin and Tessler (1989) emphasize that ruminations involve both automatic and controlled processes. For example, following a negative event such as the death of a close relative, a person may attempt to analyze the implications of this loss for his or her life and try to form new strategies and plans. At the same time the person may find that he or she is subject to images of the relative, images that appear unpredictably and that have an intrusive, disturbing quality. The authors argue that rumination involves attempts to find ways of reaching important unattained goals or attempts to find ways of reconciling oneself to not reaching those goals.

It is unlikely that this explanation of rumination provides a comprehensive account of the genesis of OCD and related disorders. Stressors appear to play only a minor role in OCD, and a characteristic feature of the symptoms of OCD is their senselessness, or the lack of relation between goals and symptoms. Advances in cognitive psychology may, however, have clinical relevance. Cognitive theories that employ cybernetic constructs, for example, may be useful in explaining the characteristic senselessness of ruminations in OCD. Thus it has been suggested that in OCD there is a persistence of high error signals or mismatch, resulting in subjective incompleteness and doubt as well as repetitive behaviors to reduce such signals (Pitman 1987a). Furthermore, cognitive theories of clinical phenomena may be useful in suggesting different methods for cognitive-behavioral therapy, and, as Josephson and Brondolo (see Chapter 11) argue, such therapy can be efficacious in the treatment of OCD and OCRDs.

Obsessive-Compulsive Disorder and Anxiety and Depression

Although the DSM classification system claims to be atheoretical, we have argued that it does embody certain theoretical assumptions. For example, in terms of the differentiation that we have drawn between OCD as on a spectrum with psychotic or personality problems, the DSM rejects this and places OCD on a spectrum with the anxiety disorders. Furthermore, the diagnostic criteria for OCD emphasize that obsessions are senseless and elicit resistance, thus differentiating them from the delusionality of psychosis and the ego-syntonicity of personality disorder. Finally, the diagnostic criteria suggest that compulsions occur in order to decrease anxiety.

These operational definitions warrant further consideration. While the DSM manuals note that overvalued ideas may occur, some studies suggest that up to 35% of patients with OCD do not regard their obsessions as senseless (Stern and Cobb 1978) and that a proportion of patients are absolutely convinced of them (Insel and Akiskal 1986). Resistance to obsessions varies a great deal (Insel and Akiskal 1986; Stern and Cobb 1978). Compulsions may take place divorced from obsessional ideas and may be experienced as involuntary and purposeless. On the other hand, others have been concerned that the worries of generalized anxiety disorder may be classified as obsessions (Mackenzie et al. 1990), or that subclinical OCD may be ignored by the DSM. The DSM-IV Task Force is presently conducting field trials with the goal of reformulating the diagnostic criteria for OCD.

The classification of OCD as an anxiety disorder also bears further consideration. Again, there are a number of arguments for and against this position. It is clear that many patients with OCD do suffer from anxiety. It may also be argued that there is some phenomenological overlap between the various anxiety disorders. Thus there appears to be some similarity between the experience of phobia and consequent avoidance, and that of obsessionality and subsequent compulsivity. Compulsive cleaning behavior, for example, can be construed as the consequence of a dirt-disease-contamination phobia (Rachman 1976). The pattern of fear and avoidance in panic disorder has also been compared with OCD, and it has been noted that agoraphobic individuals often have obsessional concerns and compulsive behaviors related to traveling (Turner et al. 1979). On the other hand, phobias and phobic avoidance generally require the presence of the feared object or situation to trigger symptomatology, whereas this is not the case in OCD. Obsessional doubts may become *more*, not less, certain with reassurance, and it has been noted that the performance of rituals may increase anxiety. Finally, when there is an increase in external stress, some OCD patients may have a decrease in symptoms (Insel 1982).

A number of studies indicate that patients with OCD are more likely to have symptoms of other anxiety disorders, as are relatives of patients with OCD (Rasmussen and Eisen 1990). Furthermore, there appears to be some overlap in neurobiological markers and therapeutic response. Thus *m*-chlorophenylpiperazine (m-CPP), a partial serotonin agonist, causes an exacerbation of OCD symptomatology (Hollander et al. 1988a; Zohar et al. 1987) in a subgroup of OCD patients and can trigger panic-like attacks (Kahn et al. 1988) in panic-prone individuals. Fluoxetine, a serotonin reuptake blocker, appears useful in the treatment of both panic disorder (Gorman et al. 1987) and OCD (Liebowitz et al. 1989). On the other hand, a variety of panicogens, including lactate (Gorman et al. 1985) and yohimbine (Rasmussen et al. 1987), do not exacerbate OCD. Furthermore, fluoxetine is effective at much lower doses and the response time is quicker in panic disorder than in OCD. Clomipramine appears to have a differential benefit over other antidepressants in the case of OCD (Leonard et al. 1988; Zohar and Insel 1987), whereas this difference is not apparent when these agents are used to treat other anxiety disorders.

Although the DSM manuals do not indicate that OCD is a mood disorder, the relationship between OCD and depression has also received some consideration. OCD was considered a variant of depression by Maudsley, and psychoanalysts have long argued that most depressive patients have obsessional personalities. Certainly, OCD is often accompanied by depression (Rasmussen and Eisen 1990). Depression, on the other hand is accompanied by ruminations that may have an obsessive nature, as well as by obsessive-compulsive symptoms (Kendell and Discipio 1970; Peselow et al. 1990; Vaughan 1976). Nevertheless, the ruminations of depression occur against the background of depressed mood and, within that context, differ from the senseless intrusion of OCD obsessions. A number of biological markers suggest similarities between OCD and depression (Insel 1983). Serotonin has long been thought to play an important role in depression (Meltzer 1990), and OCD has been found to respond to a variety of antidepressants. Nevertheless, serotonin has been more closely linked to OCD than to depression, and the specificity of the response of OCD to serotonergic medication differs from the general response to antidepressants seen in mood disorders. Again, in the case of fluoxetine, antiobsessional doses are higher and take longer to work than antidepressant doses. Furthermore, the efficacy of antidepressant medication in OCD is not dependent on the presence of coexistent depression (DeVeaugh-Geiss et al. 1988). In short, it seems that some of the links between OCD and anxiety also pertain to OCD and depression.

In summary, we would conclude that although there is some evidence for retaining the concept of OCD as an anxiety disorder, further consideration and validation are required. Alternative ways of conceptualizing (and therefore perhaps of classifying) the OCD spectrum also require exploration. In the following sections we consider the overlap between OCD and TS, trichotillomania, BDD, hypochondriasis, and eating disorders.

Obsessive-Compulsive Disorder and Tourette's Syndrome

In this section we will discuss some of the neurological and organic disorders that appear to be on a spectrum with OCD. Advances in the neurobiology of both OCD and these various disorders allow us to consider in greater depth the neurochemical and neuroanatomical substrate of the spectrum of obsessive-compulsivity.

One of the most intriguing relationships of OCD is that with Tourette's syndrome. Gilles de la Tourette's (1885) initial description of the syndrome included a patient with tics, vocalizations, and perhaps obsessions. Recent studies have confirmed this association between recurrent motor and phonic tics of TS and obsessive-compulsive symptomatology (Hollander et al. 1989b; see also Leckman, Chapter 6). The occurrence of tics in patients with OCD has also been noted (Pitman et al. 1987; Rasmussen and Tsuang 1986). Indeed, Pitman et al. (1987) found that tics were more useful in distinguishing relatives of patients with OCD from relatives of control subjects than were obsessions or compulsions.

To some extent, the ego-dystonic experience of obsessions as intrusive and senseless differentiates OCD from TS, in which tics are not necessarily perceived as intrusive and may be accompanied by a welcome release of tension. Furthermore, while compulsions are defined as purposeful and intentional and are designed to prevent discomfort or some dreaded event, tics are often purposeless and involuntary and are not generally connected with dread or prevention of some future event. Nevertheless, obsessions may become ego-syntonic, and compulsions may be felt as involuntary and need not be associated with future harm, particularly in patients with the need for perfection or symmetry. Conversely, just as obsessions may be resisted by the patient, so tics may be suppressed for a brief period of time. Also, just as compulsions often result in a reduction of anxiety, so tics result in reduced tension. The distinction between complex tics and compulsions may therefore be difficult to make.

The term "impulsions" was employed by Bender and Schilder (1940) to describe a childhood phenomenon in which there was preoccupation with a specific subject (e.g., motor cars), leading to the performance of specific actions (e.g., painting cars). Impulsions differed from obsessions and compulsions in that patients were not bothered by them. Shapiro et al. (1988) have used the term "impulsions" to describe the obsessive-compulsive–like symptoms frequently found in TS (e.g., repeated touching). Touching and symmetry behavior is more common in TS than in OCD (Pitman et al. 1987). Often there is only mild resistance to such activities, and the activities may not interfere with functioning. We would agree that while the lack of distress and dysfunction often means that these symptoms do not meet the criteria for OCD, they are a common subtype of compulsion, and like compulsions they are followed by a reduction in anxiety. We would therefore consider these activities obsessive-compulsive behaviors characteristic of subclinical OCD.

It should be noted, however, that a number of symptoms commonly seen in TS, such as echo phenomena, coprolalia, self-destructive behavior, and childhood attention-deficit disorder, are seen much less frequently in OCD (Pitman et al. 1987).

Family studies indicate a high rate of OCD and/or tics in relatives of TS patients (Comings and Comings 1987; Pauls et al. 1984, 1986) and a high rate of TS and/or tics in relatives of OCD patients (Pauls 1989; Pitman et al. 1987). These authors argue that at least a subgroup of OCD patients may represent a different manifestation of the same underlying factors that are responsible for TS and chronic multiple tic disorder.

A relationship has also been established between OCD or obsessive-compulsiveness and other movement disorders including Sydenham's chorea (Rapoport 1989), von Economo's encephalitis (Jenike 1984; Schilder 1938), Huntington's disease (Dewhurst et al. 1969), and Parkinson's disease (Menza et al. 1990). Obsessive-compulsive symptoms have been noted in various organic illnesses such as Lesch-Nyhan syndrome (Yaryura-Tobias and Neziroglu 1984) and Prader-Willi syndrome. Obsessive-compulsive symptoms have occurred in a variety of other neurological disorders, including head injury (McKeon et al. 1984), birth trauma (Capstick and Seldrup 1977), seizure disorder (Bear and Fedio 1977; Kettl and Marks 1986), brain tumors (Cambier et al. 1988), diabetes insipidus (Barton 1965), and others (Grimshaw 1964). More specifically, OCD symptoms have occurred after damage to the basal ganglia (Laplane et al. 1989) and with frontal cortical lesions (Ward 1988).

An immediate question is the underlying neurochemical and neuroanatomical basis for a link between such disorders as OCD and TS. A good deal of research is now available on neurobiological similarities and differences when OCD and TS are compared. We can begin with the neurochemical.

On the basis of cerebrospinal fluid (CSF) measurements of dopamine metabolites, exacerbation of symptoms with dopamine agonists, and treatment response to dopamine blockers in TS, and on CSF 5-hydroxyindoleacetic acid (5-HIAA), pharmacological challenges with serotonin agonists and antagonists, and therapeutic response to serotonergic medication in OCD, TS has been thought of as a disorder of dopamine function, and OCD as a disorder of serotonin function (Hollander et al. 1989b; see also Chapter 6). Nevertheless, there are a number of preclinical and clinical findings which suggest that the picture is more complex than this. On the one hand there is substantial interlinkage between serotonin and dopamine tracts (Gabay 1981). Dopaminergic agents lead to a variety of stereotypies that mimic obsessive-compulsive symptoms, and dopamine is implicated in hoarding behavior (Goodman et al. 1990). OCD does not always respond to serotonergic medication, and it turns out that if medications are highly serotonin selective, they may not lead to as good a response (Jenike et al. 1990). McDougle et al. (1990) have shown the value of dopamine blockers in the treatment of some OCD patients. Conversely, in some TS patients, CSF 5-HIAA is decreased (Butler et al. 1979; Cohen et al. 1979), and postmortem studies show decreased tryptophan and serotonin in various brain regions, including the basal ganglia (Anderson et al. 1989). Studies of serotonergic probes have not yet been undertaken in TS. Clomipramine has been useful in some TS patients (Ciprian 1980; Yaryura-Tobias and Neziroglu 1977), and fluoxetine has been shown to improve obsessions and compulsions in these patients (Riddle et al. 1990). While the neurochemistry of these disorders clearly requires further investigation to clarify the exact nature of the dysfunctions and the precise contribution of the various neurotransmitter systems (including the noradrenergic system), it is apparent that there are not only differences in the underlying neurochemistry of OCD and TS, but also important similarities.

This account may also have applicability to the relationship between OCD and other neurological and organic disorders. Thus in Parkinson's disease, a disorder in which patients are noted to be stoic, industrious, and inflexible, there is not only dopaminergic dysfunction but also serotonin involvement (Mayeux et al. 1984). In Lesch-Nyhan syndrome, which is characterized by compulsive self-mutilation, 5-hydroxytryptophan has been found useful (Mizuno and Yugari 1975; Mizuno et al. 1970), and Yaryura-Tobias and Neziroglu (1984) report that clomipramine is also useful. Although the obsessive-compulsiveness in such disorders may be more dissimilar from OCD than even the obsessive-compulsive symtomatology seen in TS, the investigation of such disorders may turn out to enhance our understanding of the neurobiology of OCD and related disorders.

Attention has also been paid to possible neuroanatomical similarities between OCD and TS that would fit with the phenomenological and neurochemical similarities. Increasing mention is made of the importance of basal ganglia and orbitofrontal cortex neurocircuitry in these disorders (Modell et al. 1989; see also Chapter 6). The association between OCD and site-specific neurological disorders supports the involvement of such pathways. Furthermore, abnormal movements and soft-sign examinations are present in OCD and TS (Hollander et al. 1989b). Neuropsychological testing and electrophysiological studies in OCD and TS indicate heterogeneity within the disorders, but suggest some similar abnormalities in the two disorders (Hollander et al. 1989b). More specific evidence lies in neuropathological studies of the striatum in TS (Chase et al. 1986). Brain imaging in OCD (Baxter 1990) and TS (Chase et al. 1984) also suggests involvement of the basal ganglia and orbitofrontal cortex. Finally, psychosurgical ablation of corresponding neurocircuitry has had therapeutic efficacy in OCD (Modell et al. 1990).

Involvement of these pathways may again be of importance in understanding the association between OCD and other organic and neurological disorders.

In summary, advances in modern neurobiology suggest that OCD is related to various organic and neurological disorders on the basis of overlapping pathogenic mechanisms. Such research contributes in turn to the way in which we think of the phenomenology of the OCD spectrum. Thus it becomes increasingly likely that we will focus on tics and other neurological signs and symptoms in OCD patients and their relatives.

Obsessive-Compulsive Disorder and the Body: Grooming, Somatoform, and Eating Disorders

The finding that obsessive-compulsiveness in a variety of different disorders may have underlying pathogenic similarities leads to a review of obsessions and compulsions that are not traditionally included under the category of OCD but appear to be phenomenologically related. In this section we will focus on ruminations and rituals that concern the body. Under this rubric we will look at trichotillomania, BDD, hypochondriasis, depersonalization disorder, and anorexia nervosa. Other obsessive-compulsive habits revolving around the body include certain forms of scratching, nail biting, oral habits, head banging, and self-mutilation (Hollander et al. 1988b; Koblenzer 1987; Primeau and Fontaine 1987).

Trichotillomania

In describing the difference between the compulsions of OCD and trichotillomania, Skodol (1989) notes that although hair pulling is associated with relief, this action may not be purposeful or closely connected with preventing or producing some future event. Patients with trichotillomania appear to have only this one symptom, rather than the multiple obsessions and compulsions often found in OCD patients (Jenike 1990). While both OCD and trichotillomania have an early onset, the sex ratio in the two disorders differs markedly, with many more females than males suffering from the latter disorder (Swedo et al. 1989a). Anecdotal findings suggest that such patients have impulsive rather than compulsive personality disorders.

Nevertheless, as Swedo (see Chapter 5) notes, there is some evidence that OCD and trichotillomania have similar underpinnings. Hair pulling is often described as ego-dystonic and is resisted. Swedo reported a preliminary family study indicating a higher-than-normal incidence of both OCD and trichotillomania in first-degree relatives of patients with trichotillomania. Brain imaging in patients with trichotillomania (Swedo et al. 1990) indicates differences from OCD patients but shows that treatment efficacy is negatively correlated with anterior cingulate and orbital frontal metabolism, a finding that corresponds with data from OCD studies. Finally, Swedo et al. (1989a) report that clomipramine is more efficacious than desipramine in treating trichotillomania. Preliminary work by Winchel et al. (1989) suggests that fluoxetine is also helpful in treating trichotillomania, although our own observations (unpublished) are that fluoxetine is often not helpful. A neuroethological model suggests that OCD and trichotillomania may involve disturbances in grooming behaviors.

Somatoform Disorders: Body Dysmorphic Disorder and Hypochondriasis

Body dysmorphic disorder is characterized by preoccupation with some imagined defect in appearance in a normal-appearing person. In hypochondriasis there is preoccupation with the fear, or the belief, of having a serious disease, in the absence of a physical evaluation of abnormality. As these are somatoform disorders, it is implied that these preoccupations are not intrusive and senseless. By definition they are not of delusional intensity. Nevertheless, in BDD, hypochondriasis, and OCD, the fixity of and resistance to the pathological thought vary greatly and may change in the individual patient over time. It is therefore possible to see a phenomenological similarity between BDD, hypochondriasis, and OCD, and to postulate that the continuum between OCD and delusional disorder is seen also in BDD and hypochondriasis. As Hollander and Phillips (see Chapter 2) and Fallon et al. (see Chapter 4) point out, both BDD patients and hypochondriacal patients may have other obsessions and compulsions, and OCD patients may have concerns about body defects or disease. Obsessive-compulsive traits may be more common in BDD (Andreasen and Bardach 1977; Thomas 1984). A number of validators, such as course, prevalence, age at onset, comorbidity, level of impairment, and sex ratio, appear to be similar in BDD and OCD (Hollander et al. 1992b). At times there may be a family history of OCD in patients with BDD (Hollander et al. 1989c). Body dysmorphic symptoms of delusional intensity have been reported to be exacerbated with marijuana (Hollander et al. 1989c), and this also has been reported secondary to cyproheptadine administration (Craven and Rodin 1987), suggesting possible serotonergic involvement. There are reports of these disorders responding to antidepressants (Jenike 1990b), and our group has found fluoxetine to be helpful in treatment of both disorders (Hollander 1991; Hollander et al. 1989c; see Chapter 4). When hypochondriasis is of delusional intensity, a dopaminergic agent may be helpful (Munro and Chmara 1982).

Depersonalization Disorder

In depersonalization disorder there are concerns about the reality of one's sense of self. As this is a dissociative disorder, it is again implied that these concerns are not intrusive and senseless. Nevertheless, as Hollander and Phillips (see Chapter 2) point out, such symptoms may well be experienced as ego-dystonic. Premorbid obsessional traits have been reported in depersonalized patients (Roth 1959; Torch 1978). Conversely, doubt has long been thought central to OCD, and

Janet emphasized the role of depersonalization in OCD (Pitman 1987b). More recently, Hollander (1990b) has noted depersonalization symptoms in OCD and panic disorder patients. Depersonalization occurs with migraine (Comfort 1982) and is exacerbated by marijuana (Szymanski 1981), suggesting the involvement of serotonin. Hollander et al. (1989a, 1990b) have suggested that depersonalization disorder responds to fluoxetine.

Anorexia Nervosa

Patients with eating disorders are classically distinguished from OCD patients in that the former have obsessions and compulsions relating to the body and to eating. The obsessions and compulsions of eating disorders are often described as more ego-syntonic than those of OCD, but once more this is a variable finding. A number of early authors conceived of anorexia as a subtype of OCD (DuBois 1949; Palmer and Jones 1939). Indeed, as Kaye et al. (see Chapter 3) note, a high proportion of eating disorder patients have other obsessions and compulsions. Conversely, some patients with OCD have concerns with the body and with eating.

Family studies indicate a high incidence of obsessive character traits in family members of anorexic patients (Crisp et al. 1974; Hecht et al. 1983; Kalucy et al. 1977), but work on familial incidence of OCD remains to be done. Some preliminary neurobiological research has attempted to explore the relationship between anorexia nervosa and OCD. Kaye et al. (see Chapter 3) report that high levels of CSF 5-HIAA are found in a subgroup of eating disorder patients, and a subgroup of OCD patients may also have increased levels of CSF 5-HIAA (Goodman et al. 1989; Insel et al. 1985; Thorén et al. 1980). Studies of behavioral and serotonergic responsivity to serotonergic agonists reveal similar patterns in patients with OCD and eating disorders (Brewerton et al. 1989; Buttinger et al. 1990; Jimerson et al. 1989; McBride et al. 1990). There are reports of the use of clomipramine (Crisp et al. 1987) and fluoxetine (Kaye et al. 1990) in the treatment of eating disorders. Nevertheless, it is not clear that the response to these medications is as specific as that seen in OCD.

Compulsivity and Impulsivity

At first glance, OCD and impulsive symptoms such as kleptomania, fire setting, self-mutilation, explosive aggression, compulsive gambling and shopping, and some patterns of sexuality and drug abuse, seem inversely related. Obsessions are experienced as intrusive, senseless, and repetitive, whereas impulsive thoughts may be ego-syntonic and unpremeditated. Compulsions are related to the avoidance of discomfort or future harm, whereas impulsive acts can be pleasurable and can result in harm. Moreover, psychodynamic theory teaches us to think of obsessive-compulsivity as a neurotic regression to anal-sadistic concerns, whereas impulsivity is conceived of as a more pathological consequence of ego and superego deficits. Nevertheless, both obsessive-compulsive and impulsive symptoms fall on a spectrum from ego-syntonic to ego-dystonic, and both types of symptoms may involve repetitive patterns. Both symptom groups may elicit resistance and result in anxiety reduction. Furthermore, many patients with OCD have aggressive thoughts, focusing on impulsive acts toward self or others. There appears to be a subgroup of OCD patients with a history of poor impulse control (Gardner and Gardner 1975; Hoehn-Saric and Barksdale 1983), or with primitive defenses (Insel 1982). In some of the OCRDs such as TS or pathological gambling, self- and other-directed impulsivity is even more apparent (Pitman et al. 1987; Yaryura-Tobias and Neziroglu 1984; see also Chapter 8). Conversely, Kernberg (1985) has noted the presence of obsessive-compulsive symptoms in impulsive borderline patients.

Cloninger (1987) has proposed that harm avoidance comprises a personality dimension that can be reliably measured. We elected to administer his Tridimensional Personality Questionnaire (TPQ) to patients who appeared to fall on the compulsive-impulsive spectrum. Fifty patients who met DSM-III criteria for OCD, TS, trichotillomania, anorexia nervosa or bulimia, or borderline personality disorder (BPD) ($n = 10$ for each group) completed the questionnaire. Results were tabulated and compared (see Table 12–1).

Harm-avoidance scores in OCD patients (mean = 26.1) were higher than in patients with OCRDs and impulsive personality disorders.

Nevertheless, harm-avoidance scores in all patient subgroups were higher than published scores of harm avoidance in control subjects (mean = 8.3; Cloninger 1987). Thus, although patients with OCD have the highest harm-avoidance scores, patients with OCD and OCRDs are more similar to one another than to control subjects on this dimension. Reward-dependence scores were lower in OCD subjects (mean = 14.9), and higher in patients with OCRDs, than in control subjects (mean = 17.4). Novelty-seeking scores in OCD patients (mean = 13.1) were similar to those of control subjects (mean = 12.9), but these scores were higher in patients with OCRDs. Relatively low reward-dependence and novelty-seeking scores in OCD patients are not inconsistent with clinical experience (i.e., OCD patients may be detached or rigid). In sum, it appears that the compulsive-impulsive spectrum cannot simply be divided into poles of high and low harm avoidance. Rather, there may be abnormal harm avoidance in the different patient groups that fall on this spectrum.

Cloninger (1987) has argued that harm avoidance reflects serotonergic function, with high harm avoidance correlating with a hyperserotonergic state. The role of serotonin in different OCRDs has been discussed at a number of points in this volume. While a subgroup of OCD patients have high CSF levels of 5-HIAA, this is not true for all patients. Administration of the serotonin agonist m-CPP to OCD patients reveals both serotonin receptor hypersensitivity (associated with behavioral exacerbation) and subsensitivity (associated with endocrine blunting) (Hollander et al. 1992a; Zohar et al. 1987). On the basis of central and peripheral measures of serotonergic

Table 12–1.   Tridimensional personality questionnaire (TPQ) scores in compulsive and impulsive patients

	Obsessive-compulsive	Tourette's syndrome	Hair pulling	Eating disorder	Borderline personality
Reward dependence	14.9	19.3	19.3	20.8	20.4
Novelty seeking	13.1	17.5	16.7	15.7	16.9
Harm avoidance	26.1	18.7	19.8	19.6	21.5

function, as well as serotonergic challenge studies, serotonin has also
been implicated in a wide variety of impulsive behaviors, with low
serotonin function correlating with high impulsivity (Brown and
Goodwin 1986; Coccaro et al. 1989; see also Chapter 9). In a pilot
study of m-CPP in patients with impulsive personality disorders, we
found that behavioral and neuroendocrine responses differed from
those of OCD patients. Thus, while there is some support for
Cloninger's hypothesis, the biochemistry of compulsivity and impulsivity appears to be complex.

The role of serotonergic medications in the treatment of the
OCRDs has also been mentioned in many chapters. Fenfluramine
treatment, for example, may be helpful in decreasing suicidal ideation
(Meyendorff et al. 1986) and OCD symptoms (Hollander et al. 1990a).
Serotonin reuptake blockers may be useful in the treatment of both
OCD and impulsivity (see Chapter 9), and there are case reports of
the response of kleptomania, self-mutilation, and sexual compulsivity
to these medications (Hollander et al. 1988b; Levy 1990; see also
Chapter 7).

Several possibilities exist. Increased serotonergic function in OCD
may correlate inversely with impulsivity. This is supported by the
idea that compulsive patients differ from impulsive patients in their
focus on harm avoidance. This might account for anecdotal reports
of decreased obsessive-compulsivity but increased impulsive aggression during fluoxetine treatment of OCD. On the other hand, low
serotonin function in OCD may lead to increased impulsivity. This
would explain the subgroup of impulsive aggression in OCD and
related disorders. Leckman et al. (1990) reported low levels of CSF
5-HIAA in two patients with aggressive obsessions. A third alternative
is that a variety of receptor changes occur in OCD and that in some
patients the receptor profile overlaps with that seen in impulsive
patients.

The neurobiological basis for the link between OCD and impulsivity may also be investigated from a neuroanatomical viewpoint.
Laplane et al. (1989) reported a number of patients with bilateral
basal ganglia lesions who manifest obsessive-compulsive symptoms
as well as frontal-lobe syndrome, classically reported as characterized
by impulse dyscontrol. Modell et al. (1990) have argued that or-

bitofrontal cortex and basal ganglia neurocircuitry may also be central in alcoholism, a disorder that is typically conceived of as impulsive.

Conclusions

We have characterized several spectrums of OCD. OCD has been discussed in relation to delusions and obsessive-compulsive personality, anxiety and depression, disorders of grooming and the body, and impulsivity. We have indicated not only that there is some degree of phenomenological overlap between OCD and these disorders, but also that there is evidence of an overlap in pathogenic mechanisms. Several nosologic, clinical, and research implications are apparent.

Our review indicates that the current classification of OCD perhaps overemphasizes the link between OCD and anxiety and downplays the relationships between OCD and its related disorders. Operational criteria for obsessions and compulsions may also neglect the delusional and subclinical dimensions of OCD symptoms. Further consideration ought to be given to making the links between the various OCRDs more explicit in DSM-IV. Hopefully, the current DSM-IV field trials will help in the revision of the diagnostic criteria for OCD.

A careful history of tics, physical illness, body concerns, and impulsivity in patients and family should be taken in OCD and its related disorders. In treating OCRDs, consideration should be given to medications that have proven useful in treating OCD.

Further research on the relationships of OCD to its related disorders is required. These relationships may be investigated using phenomenological studies, family data, neurochemical and neuroanatomical studies, and pharmacotherapeutic dissection. Pharmacological challenges and brain imaging studies appear to be particularly promising methodologies for understanding the neurobiology of the OCD spectrum. Ultimately, family studies using the methods of molecular genetics may lead to even more detailed knowledge. Exploration of the spectrums of OCD will in turn contribute to our understanding of OCD and will lead to new ways of characterizing this important and complex disorder.

References

American Psychiatric Association: Diagnostic and Statistical Manual of Mental Disorders, 3rd Edition. Washington, DC, American Psychiatric Association, 1980

American Psychiatric Association: Diagnostic and Statistical Manual of Mental Disorders, 3rd Edition, Revised. Washington, DC, American Psychiatric Association, 1987

Anderson GM, Leckman JF, Riddle MA, et al: Recent neurochemical research on Tourette's syndrome. Paper presented at the Regional Congress on Biological Aspects of Nonpsychotic Disorder, World Federation of Societies of Biological Psychiatry, Jerusalem, 1989

Andreasen NC, Bardach J: Dysmorphophobia: symptom or disease? Am J Psychiatry 134:673–676, 1977

Barton R: Diabetes insipidus and obsessional neurosis: a syndrome. Lancet 1:133–135, 1965

Baxter LR: Brain imaging as a tool in establishing a theory of brain pathology in obsessive compulsive disorder. J Clin Psychiatry 51 (no 2, suppl):22–25, 1990

Baer L, Jenike MA, Ricciardi JN, et al: Standardized assessment of personality disorders in obsessive-compulsive disorder. Arch Gen Psychiatry 47:826–830, 1990

Bear DM, Fedio P: Quantitative analysis of interictal behavior in temporal lobe epilepsy. Arch Neurol 34:454–467, 1977

Bender L, Schilder P: Impulsions: a specific disorder of the behavior of children. Archives of Neurology and Psychiatry 44:990–1008, 1940

Black A: The natural history of obsessional neurosis, in Obsessional States. Edited by Beech HR. London, Methuen, 1974, pp 1–23

Brewerton T, Murphy D, Jimerson DC: A comparison of neuroendocrine responses to L-TRP and m-CPP in bulimics and controls. Biol Psychiatry 25 (no 7A, suppl):19A, 1989

Brown GL, Goodwin FK: Cerebrospinal fluid correlates of suicide attempts and aggression. Ann N Y Acad Sci 487:175–188, 1986

Butler IJ, Koslow SH, Seifert WE Jr, et al: Biogenic amine metabolism in Tourette syndrome. Ann Neurol 6:37–39, 1979

Buttinger K, Hollander E, Walsh BT: m-CPP challenges in anorexia nervosa. Paper presented at the 143rd annual meeting of the American Psychiatric Association, New York, May 1990

Cambier J, Masson C, Benammou S, et al: La graphomanie, activité graphique compulsive manifestation d'un gliome fronto-calleux. Rev Neurol (Paris) 144:158–164, 1988

Capstick N, Seldrup U: Obsessional states: a study in the relationship between abnormalities occurring at birth and subsequent development of obsessional symptoms. Acta Psychiatr Scand 56:427–439, 1977

Chase TN, Foster NL, Fedio P, et al: Gilles de la Tourette syndrome: studies with the fluorine-18–labeled fluorodeoxyglucose positron emission tomographic method. Ann Neurol 15(suppl):S175, 1984

Chase TN, Geoffrey V, Gillespie M, et al: Structural and functional studies of Gilles de la Tourette syndrome. Rev Neurol (Paris) 142:851–855, 1986

Ciprian J: Three cases of Gilles de la Tourette's syndrome. Treatment with chlorimipramine: a preliminary report. Journal of Orthomolecular Psychiatry 9:116–120, 1980

Cloninger CR: A systematic method for clinical description and classification of personality variants: a proposal. Arch Gen Psychiatry 44:573–588, 1987

Coccaro EF, Siever LJ, Klar HM, et al: Serotonergic studies in patients with affective and personality disorders: correlations with suicidal and impulsive aggressive behavior. Arch Gen Psychiatry 46:587–599, 1989

Cohen DJ, Shaywitz BA, Young JG, et al: Central biogenic amine metabolism in children with the syndrome of chronic multiple tics of Gilles de la Tourette: norepinephrine, serotonin, and dopamine. Journal of the American Academy of Child Psychiatry 18:320–341, 1979

Comfort A: Out-of-body experiences and migraine (letter). Am J Psychiatry 139:1379–1380, 1982

Comings DE, Comings BG: Hereditary agoraphobia and obsessive-compulsive behaviour in relatives of patients with Gilles de la Tourette's syndrome. Br J Psychiatry 151:195–199, 1987

Craven JL, Rodin GM: Cyproheptadine dependence associated with an atypical somatoform disorder. Can J Psychiatry 32:143–145, 1987

Crisp AH, Harding B, McGuinness B: Anorexia nervosa. Psychoneurotic characteristics of parents: relationship to prognosis, a quantitative study. J Psychosom Res 18:167–173, 1974

Crisp AH, Lacey JH, Crutchfield M: Clomipramine and 'drive' in people with anorexia nervosa: an in-patient study. Br J Psychiatry 150:355–358, 1987

DeVeaugh-Geiss J, Katz R, Landau P, et al: A multicenter trial of Anafranil in obsessive compulsive disorder. Paper presented at the 141st annual meeting of the American Psychiatric Association, Montreal, May 1988

Dewhurst K, Oliver J, Trick KLK, et al: Neuro-psychiatric aspects of Huntington's disease. Confinia Neurologica 31:258–268, 1969

Dubois FS: Compulsion neurosis with cachexia (anorexia nervosa). Am J
    Psychiatry 106:107–115, 1949–1950

Fenton W, McGlashan T: Obsessional/compulsive symptoms in schizophrenia,
    in New Research Program and Abstracts, the 138th annual meeting of the
    American Psychiatric Association, Dallas, TX, May 1985, NR12, p 24

Frances A: Categorical and dimensional systems of personality diagnosis: a
    comparison. Compr Psychiatry 23:516–527, 1982

Gabay S: Serotonergic-dopaminergic interactions: implications for hyper-
    kinetic disorders, in Advances in Experimental Medicine and Biology.
    Edited by Haber B, Gabay S, Issidorides MR, et al. New York, Plenum,
    1981, pp 285–291

Gardner AR, Gardner AJ: Self-mutilation, obsessionality and narcissism. Br
    J Psychiatry 127:127–132, 1975

Gilles de la Tourette: Étude sur une affection nerveuse caractérisée par de
    l'incoordination motrice accompagnée d'echolalie et de coprolalie. Arch
    Neurol 9:19–42, 158–200, 1885

Goodman WK, Price LH, Anderson GM, et al: Drug response and obsessive
    compulsive disorder subtypes. Paper presented at the 142nd annual
    meeting of the American Psychiatric Association, San Francisco, CA, May
    1989

Goodman WK, McDougle CJ, Price LH, et al: Beyond the serotonin
    hypothesis: a role for dopamine in some forms of obsessive-compulsive
    disorder? J Clin Psychiatry 51 (no 8, suppl):36–43, 1990

Goodwin DW, Guze SB, Robins E: Follow-up studies in obsessional
    neurosis. Arch Gen Psychiatry 20:182–187, 1969

Gorman J, Leibowitz M, Fyer A, et al: Lactate infusions in obsessive-com-
    pulsive disorder. Am J Psychiatry 142:864–866, 1985

Gorman JM, Liebowitz MR, Fyer AJ, et al: An open trial of fluoxetine in the
    treatment of panic attacks. J Clin Psychopharmacol 7:329–332, 1987

Grimshaw L: Obsessional disorder and neurological illness. J Neurol Neu-
    rosurg Psychiatry 27:229, 1964

Hecht AM, Fichter M, Postpischil P: Obsessive-compulsive neurosis and
    anorexia nervosa. International Journal of Eating Disorders 2:69–77, 1983

Hoehn-Saric R, Barksdale VC: Impulsiveness in obsessive-compulsive pa-
    tients. Br J Psychiatry 143:177–182, 1983

Hollander E, Fay M, Cohen B, et al: Serotonergic and noradrenergic
    sensitivity in obsessive-compulsive disorder: behavioral findings. Am J
    Psychiatry 145:1015–1017, 1988a

Hollander E, Papp L, Campeas R, et al: More on self mutilation and obsessive
    compulsive disorder (letter). Can J Psychiatry 33:675, 1988b

Hollander E, Fairbanks J, DeCaria C, et al: Pharmacological dissection of panic and depersonalization (letter). Am J Psychiatry 146:402, 1989a

Hollander E, Liebowitz MR, DeCaria CM: Conceptual and methodological issues in studies of obsessive-compulsive and Tourette's disorders. Psychiatr Dev 7:267–296, 1989b

Hollander E, Liebowitz MR, Winchel R, et al: Treatment of body-dysmorphic disorder with serotonin reuptake blockers. Am J Psychiatry 146:768–770, 1989c

Hollander E, DeCaria CM, Schneier FR, et al: Fenfluramine augmentation of serotonin reuptake blockade antiobsessional treatment. J Clin Psychiatry 51:119–123, 1990a

Hollander E, Liebowitz MR, DeCaria C, et al: Treatment of depersonalization with serotonin reuptake blockers. J Clin Psychopharmacol 10:200–203, 1990b

Hollander E: Serotonergic drugs and the treatment of disorders related to obsessive-compulsive disorders, in Current Treatments of Obsessive-Compulsive Disorder. Edited by Pato MT, Zohar J. Washington, DC, American Psychiatric Press, 1991, pp 173–191

Hollander E, DeCaria C, Nitescu A, et al: Serotonergic function in obsessive-compulsive disorder: behavioral and neuroendocrine responses to oral m-chlorophenylpiperazine and fenfluramine in patients and healthy volunteers. Arch Gen Psychiatry 49:21–28, 1992a

Hollander E, Neville D, Frenkel M, et al: Body dysmorphic disorder: diagnostic issues and related disorders. Psychosomatics 33:156–165, 1992b

Insel TR: Obsessive compulsive disorder—five clinical questions and a suggested approach. Compr Psychiatry 23:241–251, 1982

Insel TR: Biological markers and obsessive compulsive and affective disorders. J Psychiatr Res 18:407–423, 1983

Insel TR, Akiskal HS: Obsessive-compulsive disorder with psychotic features: a phenomenologic analysis. Am J Psychiatry 143:1527–1533, 1986

Insel TR, Mueller EA, Alterman I, et al: Obsessive-compulsive disorder and serotonin: is there a connection? Biol Psychiatry 20:1174–1188, 1985

Jenike MA: Obsessive-compulsive disorder: a question of a neurologic lesion. Compr Psychiatry 25:298–304, 1984

Jenike MA: Illnesses related to obsessive-compulsive disorder, in Obsessive-Compulsive Disorders: Theory and Management, 2nd Edition. Edited by Jenike MA, Baer LB, Minichiello WE. Chicago, IL, Year Book Medical, 1990, pp 39–60

Jenike MA, Hyman S, Baer L, et al: A controlled trial of fluvoxamine in obsessive-compulsive disorder: implications for a serotonergic theory. Am J Psychiatry 147:1209–1215, 1990

Jimerson DC, Lesem MD, Kaye WH, et al: Serotonin and symptom severity in eating disorders. Biol Psychiatry 25(suppl):141A, 1989

Joffe RT, Swinson RP, Regan JJ: Personality features of obsessive-compulsive disorder. Am J Psychiatry 145:1127–1129, 1988

Kahn RS, Wetzler S, van Praag HM, et al: Neuroendocrine evidence for serotonin receptor hypersensitivity in panic disorder. Psychopharmacology (Berlin) 96:360–364, 1988

Kalucy RS, Crisp AH, Harding B: A study of 56 families with anorexia nervosa. Br J Med Psychol 50:381–395, 1977

Kaye W, Wletzin T, Hsu G: An open trial of fluoxetine in adolescent weight-recovered anorexics. Paper presented at the annual meeting of the American College of Neuropsychopharmacology, San Juan, Puerto Rico, 1990

Kendell RE: The Role of Diagnosis in Psychiatry, Oxford, UK, Blackwell, 1975

Kendell RE, Discipio WJ: Obsessional symptoms and obsessional personality traits in patients with depressive illness. Psychol Med 1:65–72, 1970

Kernberg O: Borderline Conditions and Pathological Narcissism. New York, Jason Aronson, 1985

Kettl PA, Marks IM: Neurological factors in obsessive compulsive disorder: two case reports and a review of the literature. Br J Psychiatry 149:315–319, 1986

Koblenzer CS: Psychocutaneous Disease. New York, Grune & Stratton, 1987

Laplane D, Levasseur M, Pillon B, et al: Obsessive-compulsive and other behavioral changes with bilateral basal ganglia lesions. Brain 112:699–725, 1989

Leckman JF, Goodman WK, Riddle MA, et al: Low CSF 5-HIAA and obsessions of violence: report of two cases. Psychiatry Res 33:95–99, 1990

Leonard H, Swedo S, Rapoport JL, et al: Treatment of childhood obsessive compulsive disorder with clomipramine and desmethylimipramine: a double-blind crossover comparison. Psychopharmacol Bull 24:93–95, 1988

Levy R: Is obsessive-compulsive disorder (OCD) the basis for several pathological states? Paper presented at the annual meeting of the American Academy of Clinical Psychiatry, October 1990

Liebowitz MR, Hollander E, Schneier F, et al: Fluoxetine treatment of obsessive-compulsive disorder: an open clinical trial. J Clin Psychopharmacol 9:423–427, 1989

Mackenzie TB, Christenson G, Kroll J: Obsession or worry (letter)? Am J Psychiatry 147:1573, 1990

Martin LL, Tesser A: Toward a motivational and structural theory of ruminative thought, in Unintended Thought. Edited by Uleman JS, Bargh JA. New York, Guilford, 1989, pp 306–326

Mayeux R, Stern Y, Cote L, et al: Altered serotonin metabolism in depressed patients with Parkinson's disease. Neurology 34:642–646, 1984

McBride PA, Anderson GM, Khait VD, et al: Serotonergic responsivity in eating disorders. Paper presented at the annual meeting of the American College of Neuropsychopharmacology, San Juan, Puerto Rico, 1990

McDougle CJ, Goodman WK, Price LH, et al: Neuroleptic addition in fluvoxamine-refractory obsessive-compulsive disorder. Am J Psychiatry 147:652–654, 1990

McKeon J, McGuffin P, Robinson P: Obsessive-compulsive neurosis following head injury: a report of four cases. Br J Psychiatry 144:190–192, 1984

Meltzer HY: Role of serotonin in depression. Ann N Y Acad Sci 600:486–500, 1990

Menza MA, Forman NE, Goldstein HS, et al: Parkinson's disease, personality, and dopamine. Journal of Neuropsychiatry and Clinical Neurosciences 2:282–287, 1990

Meyendorff E, Jain A, Träskman-Bendz L, et al: The effects of fenfluramine on suicidal behavior. Psychopharmacol Bull 22:155–159, 1986

Mizuno T, Yugari Y: Prophylactic effect of L-5-hydroxytryptophan on self-mutilation in the Lesch-Nyhan syndrome. Neuropaediatrie 6:13–23, 1975

Mizuno T, Segawa M, Kurumada T, et al: Clinical and therapeutic aspects of the Lesch-Nyhan syndrome in Japanese children. Neuropaediatrie 2:38–52, 1970

Modell JG, Mountz JM, Curtis GC, et al: Neurophysiologic dysfunction in basal ganglia/limbic striatal and thalamocortical circuits as a pathogenetic mechanism of obsessive-compulsive disorder. Journal of Neuropsychiatry and Clinical Neurosciences 1:27–36, 1989

Modell JG, Mountz JM, Beresford TP: Basal ganglia/limbic striatal and thalamocortical involvement in craving and loss of control in alcoholism. Journal of Neuropsychiatry and Clinical Neurosciences 2:123–144, 1990

Munro A, Chmara J: Monosymptomatic hypochondriacal psychosis: a diagnostic checklist based on 50 cases of the disorder. Can J Psychiatry 27:374–376, 1982

Palmer HD, Jones MS: Anorexia nervosa as a manifestation of compulsion neurosis: a study of psychogenic factors. Archives of Neurology and Psychiatry 41:856–860, 1939

Pauls DL: The familial relationship of obsessive compulsive disorder and Tourette's syndrome. Paper presented at the 142nd annual meeting of the American Psychiatric Association, San Francisco, CA, May 1989

Pauls DL, Kruger SD, Leckman JF, et al: The risk of Tourette's syndrome and chronic multiple tics among relatives of Tourette's syndrome patients obtained by direct interview. Journal of the American Academy of Child Psychiatry 23:134–137, 1984

Pauls DL, Towbin KE, Leckman JF, et al: Gilles de la Tourette's syndrome and obsessive-compulsive disorder: evidence supporting a genetic relationship. Arch Gen Psychiatry 43:1180–1182, 1986

Peselow ED, DiFiglia C, Fieve RR: Obsessive-compulsive symptoms in patients with major depression: frequency and response to antidepressant treatment. Paper presented at the annual meeting of the American College of Neurpsychopharmacology, San Juan, Puerto Rico, 1990

Pitman RK: A cybernetic model of obsessive-compulsive psychopathology. Compr Psychiatry 28:334–343, 1987a

Pitman RK: Pierre Janet on obsessive-compulsive disorder (1903): review and commentary. Arch Gen Psychiatry 44:226–232, 1987b

Pitman RK, Green RC, Jenike MA, et al: Clinical comparison of Tourette's disorder and obsessive-compulsive disorder. Am J Psychiatry 144:1166–1171, 1987

Pollack JM: Obsessive-compulsive personality: a review. Psychol Bull 86:225–241, 1979

Pollack JM: Relationship of obsessive-compulsive personality to obsessive-compulsive disorder: a review of the literature. J Psychol 121:137–148, 1987

Primeau F, Fontaine R: Obsessive disorder with self-mutilation: a subgroup responsive to pharmacotherapy. Can J Psychiatry 32:699–701, 1987

Rachman S: The modification of obsessions: a new formulation. Behav Res Ther 14:437–443, 1976

Rachman S, Da Silva P: Abnormal and normal obsessions. Behav Res Ther 16:233–248, 1978

Rapoport JL: The biology of obsessions and compulsions. Sci Am 3:83–89, 1989

Rasmussen SA, Eisen JL: Epidemiological and clinical features of obsessive-compulsive disorder, in Obsessive-Compulsive Disorders: Theory and Management, 2nd Edition. Edited by Jenike MA, Baer LB, Minichiello WE. Chicago, IL, Year Book Medical, 1990

Rassmussen SA, Tsuang MT: Clinical characteristics and family history in DSM-III obsessive-compulsive disorder. Am J Psychiatry 143:317–322, 1986

Rasmussen SA, Goodman WK, Woods SW, et al: Effects of yohimbine in obsessive-compulsive disorder. Psychopharmacology (Berlin) 93:308–313, 1987

Reed G: Obsessional personality disorder and remembering. Br J Psychiatry 130:177–183, 1977

Riddle MA, Hardin MT, King R, et al: Fluoxetine treatment of children and adolescents with Tourette's and obsessive compulsive disorders: preliminary clinical experience. J Am Acad Child Adolesc Psychiatry 29:45–48, 1990

Rosen I: The clinical significance of obsessions in schizophrenia. Journal of Mental Science 103:773–785, 1957

Rosen W, Hollander E, Stannick V, et al: Task performance variables in obsessive-compulsive disorder. J Clin Neuropsychol 10:73, 1988

Roth M: The phobic anxiety depersonalization sydrome. Journal of Neuropsychiatry 1:293–306, 1959

Salzman L: Obsessional Personality, New York, Science House, 1968

Schilder P: The organic background of obsessions and compulsions. Am J Psychiatry 94:1397–1416, 1938

Shapiro AK, Shapiro ES, Young JG, et al: Gilles de la Tourette Syndrome, 2nd Edition. New York, Raven, 1988

Skodol AE: Problems in Differential Diagnosis: From DSM-III to DSM-III-R in Clinical Practice. Washington, DC, American Psychiatric Press, 1989

Stern RS, Cobb JP: Phenomenology of obsessive-compulsive neurosis. Br J Psychiatry 132:233–239, 1978

Swedo SE, Leonard HL, Rapoport JL, et al: A double-blind comparison of clomipramine and desipramine in the treatment of trichotillomania (hair pulling). N Engl J Med 321:497–501, 1989a

Swedo SE, Rapoport JL, Leonard H, et al: Obsessive-compulsive disorder in children and adolescents: clinical phenomenology of 70 consecutive cases. Arch Gen Psychiatry 46:335–341, 1989b

Swedo SE, Grady C, Leonard HL: PET examination of women with trichotillomania. Paper presented at the annual meeting of the American College of Neuropsychopharmacology, San Juan, Puerto Rico, 1990

Szymanski HV: Prolonged depersonalization after marijuana use. Am J Psychiatry 138:231–233, 1981

Thomas CS: Dysmorphophobia: a question of definition. Br J Psychiatry 144:513–516, 1984

Thorén P, Åsberg M, Bertilsson L, et al: Clomipramine treatment of obsessive-compulsive disorder, II: biochemical aspects. Arch Gen Psychiatry 37:1289–1294, 1980

Torch E: Review of the relationship between obsession and depersonalization. Acta Psychiatr Scand 58:191–198, 1978

Turner SM, Hersen M, Bellack AS, et al: Behavioral treatment of obsessive-compulsive neurosis. Behav Res Ther 17:95–106, 1979

Vaughan M: The relationships between obsessional personality, obsession in depression, and symptoms of depression. Br J Psychiatry 129:36–39, 1976

Ward CD: Transient feelings of compulsion caused by hemispheric lesions: three cases. J Neurol Neurosurg Psychiatry 51:266–268, 1988

Winchel R, Stanley B, Guido J: A pilot study of fluoxetine for trichotillomania. Paper presented at the 28th annual meeting of the American College of Neuropsychopharmacology, Maui, HI, 1989

Yaryura-Tobias JA, Neziroglu FA: Gilles de la Tourette syndrome: a new clinico-therapeutic approach. Progress in Neuro-psychopharmacology 1:335–338, 1977

Yaryura-Tobias JA, Neziroglu FA: Obsessive-Compulsive Disorders: Pathogenesis, Diagnosis, Treatment. New York, Marcel Dekker, 1984

Zohar J, Insel TR: Obsessive-compulsive disorder: psychobiological approaches to diagnosis, treatment, and pathophysiology. Biol Psychiatry 22:667–687, 1987

Zohar J, Mueller A, Insel TR, et al: Serotonergic responsivity in obsessive-compulsive disorder: comparison of patients and healthy controls. Arch Gen Psychiatry 44:946–951, 1987

Index

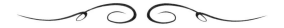